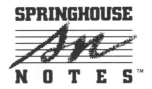

**SPRINGHOUSE**

**N O T E S** ™

# MENTAL HEALTH AND PSYCHIATRIC NURSING

═══ **SECOND EDITION** ═══

D1127908

**Margaret P. Benner, RN, PhD, CS**
Staff Nurse
Psychiatric Admissions and Evaluation Unit
Coatesville Veterans' Administration Medical Center
Coatesville, Pennsylvania

Springhouse Corporation
Springhouse, Pennsylvania

# Staff

**Executive Director, Editorial**
Stanley Loeb

**Director of Trade and Textbooks**
Minnie B. Rose, RN, BSN, MEd

**Art Director**
John Hubbard

**Clinical Consultant**
Maryann Foley, RN, BSN

**Editors**
David Moreau, Claudia Allen

**Copy Editor**
Pamela Wingrod

**Designers**
Stephanie Peters (associate art director),
Jacalyn Facciolo

**Typography**
David Kosten (director), Diane Paluba (manager),
Elizabeth Bergman, Joyce Rossi Biletz, Phyllis
Marron, Robin Mayer, Valerie L. Rosenberger

**Manufacturing**
Deborah Meiris (manager), T.A. Landis, Anna
Brindisi

**Library of Congress Cataloging-in-Publication Data**

Benner, Margaret P.
 Mental health and psychiatric nursing/
Margaret P. Benner.—2nd ed.
 p. cm. — (Springhouse notes)
 Includes bibliographical references and index.
 1. Psychiatric nursing  I. Title.  II. Series.
 [DNLM: 1. Mental Disorders—nursing—
outlines. 2. Psychiatric Nursing—outlines.  WY
18 B469m]
RC440.B38     1993
610.73'68—dc20
DNLM/DLC                                    92-2184
ISBN 0-87434-487-5                              CIP

# Contents

Advisory Board and Reviewer ................... v

How to Use Springhouse Notes ................ vi

1. Conceptual Models of Psychiatric Care ........ 1

2. Roles and Functions of Psychiatric
   Nurses ................................. 9

3. Stress and Psychophysiologic Disorders ...... 18

4. Dying and Grieving ............................ 25

5. Alterations in Self-Concept ..................... 32

6. Anxiety ................................. 39

7. Disordered Behaviors Associated with
   Anxiety ................................. 47

8. Mood Disorders .............................. 55

9. Suicide ................................. 65

10. Alteration in Thought and Perception:
    Schizophrenia ..................................... 75

11. Disruptions in Social Relatedness:
    Personality Disorders ........................... 87

12. Substance Abuse ............................ 94

13. Anger ................................. 108

14. Assaultive Behavior ........................... 115

15. Family Abuse and Violence .................... 124

16. Treatment Modalities and the Role of the
    Psychiatric Nurse .............................. 133

Appendix A: Glossary ........................... 142

Appendix B: Answers to Study
Questions ......................................... 149

Appendix C: ANA Classification of Human
Responses of Concern for Psychiatric
Mental Health Nursing Practice .............. 157

Selected References ............................ 162

Index ............................................. 163

# Advisory Board and Reviewer

v

# How to Use Springhouse Notes

Springhouse Notes is a multi-volume study guide series developed especially for nursing students. Each volume provides essential course material in an outline format, enabling the student to review the information efficiently.

Special features recur throughout the book to make the information accessible and easy to remember. *Learning objectives* begin each chapter, encouraging the student to evaluate knowledge before and after study. Next, within the outlined text, *key points* are highlighted in shaded blocks to facilitate a quick review of critical information. Key points may include cardinal signs and symptoms, current theories, important steps in a nursing procedure, critical assessment findings, crucial nursing interventions, or successful therapies and treatments. *Points to remember* summarize each chapter's major themes. *Study questions* then offer another opportunity to review material and assess knowledge gained before moving on to new information. Difficult, frequently used, or sometimes misunderstood terms (indicated by small capital letters in the outline) are gathered at the end of each chapter and defined in the *glossary*, Appendix A; answers to the study questions appear in Appendix B.

The Springhouse Notes volumes are designed as learning tools, not as primary information sources. When read conscientiously as a supplement to class attendance and textbook reading, Springhouse Notes can enhance understanding and help improve test scores and final grades.

## CHAPTER 1

# Conceptual Models of Psychiatric Care

## Learning objectives

Check off the following items once you've mastered them:

☐ Discuss key aspects of the eight theoretical models of personality and behavior.

☐ Identify each model's major theorists.

☐ Compare and contrast the underlying assumptions of each model.

☐ Describe the roles of the therapist and the client within each model.

## I. Behavioral model

A. General comments
  1. Rooted in psychology and neurophysiology, the behavioral model is associated with Pavlov, B.F. Skinner, and J. Wolpe
  2. The behavioral model regards symptoms as clusters of learned behaviors that persist because they are rewarded

B. Assumptions and key ideas
  1. Humans are complex animals
  2. The self is viewed as an individual's observable behavior
  3. Behavior is what an organism does
  4. People are shaped by elements in the environment
  5. The self is the structure of stimulus-response chains of habit
  6. Deviations occur when undesirable behavior is reinforced
  7. All behavior is learned

C. Therapeutic process
  1. The therapist's primary goal is to determine which client behaviors should be changed and how
  2. The therapist helps effect change of undesirable behaviors
  3. Major treatments include DESENSITIZATION, OPERANT CONDITIONING, COUNTER-CONDITIONING, AVERSION THERAPY, and TOKEN ECONOMY SYSTEM
  4. The client, as learner, must practice uncomfortable behaviors

## II. Existential model

A. General comments
  1. This model was influenced by EXISTENTIALISM, as found in the philosophical works of Sartre, Kierkegaard, and Heidegger
  2. Contemporary theorists include Frederick Perls, William Glasser, Albert Ellis, Carl Rogers, and R.D. Laing

B. Assumptions and key ideas
  1. Therapy focuses on the present
  2. Humans possess the freedom to realize their potential
  3. People act and are acted upon
  4. Behavior is mediated by self-awareness
  5. Self-awareness is modified by social interactions
  6. Deviations result when an individual is alienated from the self or the environment
  7. Lack of self-awareness prevents participation in authentic relationships

C. Therapeutic process
  1. Major treatments include GESTALT, RATIONAL-EMOTIVE, REALITY, and ENCOUNTER GROUP therapies
  2. Therapy attempts to return the client to an authentic awareness of being

3. Therapy focuses on the encounter between the client and the therapist
4. The therapist and the client are equal in their common humanity
5. The therapist acts as a guide, discouraging the client's dependence on the therapist

# III. Interpersonal model

A. General comments
  1. The interpersonal model is associated with Harry Stack Sullivan
  2. This model focuses on interactive aspects of behavior and development

B. Assumptions and key ideas
  1. Behavior is situationally produced and evolves within the context of interpersonal relationships
  2. Frequently motivated by anxiety, behavior is based on the drives for satisfaction and security
  3. Personality is an enduring pattern of interpersonal relationships
  4. People use selective inattention to defend against interpersonal anxiety
  5. The self-system resists change and consists of the "good me," the "bad me," and the "not me"
  6. Interpersonal development occurs in six phases
     a. Infancy (ages 1 to 2)
     b. Childhood (ages 2 to 6)
     c. Juvenile (ages 6 to 9)
     d. Preadolescence (ages 9 to 12)
     e. Early adolescence (ages 12 to 15)
     f. Late adolescence (ages 15 to 21)

C. Therapeutic process
  1. The therapist and the client review the client's life to explore progress through developmental stages
  2. Successful treatment depends on a healthy client-therapist relationship
  3. Therapy involves reeducation; the therapist encourages the client to learn more successful styles of relating
  4. The therapist's role is that of participant-observer

# IV. Medical model

A. General comments
  1. The medical model is based on the physician-client relationship
  2. The primary focus is on the diagnosis of mental illness
  3. The physician uses the diagnosis to define treatment

B. Assumptions and key ideas
  1. Deviant behavior reflects a central nervous system disorder
  2. Environmental and social factors may precipitate illness or predispose a client to it

C. Therapeutic process
1. The physician examines the client and diagnoses the illness, recording and classifying the diagnosis according to the American Psychiatric Association's *Diagnostic and Statistical Manual of Mental Disorders, Third Edition, Revised (DSM-III-R)*
2. The physician then prescribes treatment based on the diagnosis
3. Therapy focuses on promoting the client's trust, which fosters compliance with treatment
4. The client's role is that of a sick individual who must work to get well

## V. Biogenic model

A. General comments
1. The biogenic model has been influenced by scientific investigations into the neuroanatomy and physiology of the brain
2. The biogenic model examines biological factors that influence behavior
   a. Body types (ectomorph, endomorph, mesomorph)
   b. Genetics (heredity)
   c. Chemical factors (catecholamines, norepinephrine)
   d. Biological rhythms

B. Assumptions and key ideas
1. Body types correlate with personality traits and susceptibility to mental disorders
   a. Ectomorph – associated with schizophrenia
   b. Endomorph – linked with bipolar disorders
2. Heredity and the environment interact, causing a genetic predisposition to mental disorders
3. Chemical imbalances may be related to mental disorders
   a. Schizophrenia – associated with a defective TRANSMETHYLATION of catecholamines
   b. Depression – linked with norepinephrine deficits
   c. Mania – related to excess norepinephrine
4. Biological rhythms may affect physical and psychological well-being; this may explain the etiology of episodic or cyclical mental disorders

C. Therapeutic process
1. Characteristics of therapy are similar to those of the medical model
2. The biogenic model favors somatic treatments, such as PSYCHOSURGERY, electroconvulsive therapy, and medications

## VI. Nursing models

A. General comments
1. No universally accepted model exists; nursing theorists include H. Peplau (Interpersonal), D. Orem (Self-care), C. Roy (Adaptation), I. King (Systems), and M. Rogers (Unitary Man)
2. All nursing models incorporate a HOLISTIC approach

    3. Nursing models focus on the client's biological, psychological, and sociocultural needs and on the nurse's caring functions

B. Assumptions and key ideas
    1. Basic concepts include person, the environment, and health
    2. Of primary importance is an individual's response to actual or potential health problems
    3. Viewed on a continuum, client behavior results from a combination of predisposing factors and precipitating STRESSORS

C. Therapeutic process
    1. The client's needs are the focus of a therapeutic nurse-client relationship
    2. The client and the nurse collaborate, with the nurse acting as client advocate
    3. The nurse intervenes at any point along the health-illness continuum
    4. The nursing process defines care, and nursing care goals are based on nursing diagnoses established by the North American Nursing Diagnosis Association (NANDA); diagnoses specific to psychiatric nursing are currently being reviewed for acceptance by NANDA (see Appendix C, page 157)
    5. Significant nursing functions include coordinating health care, applying comfort measures to ease pain, and helping the client maximize capabilities

# VII. Psychoanalytic model

A. General comments
    1. Sigmund Freud is the accepted father of this model
    2. Sexuality is a central concept in development
    3. Disruptive behavior in adults originates in earlier developmental stages
    4. Study of NEUROTIC BEHAVIOR led to this theory

B. Assumptions and key ideas
    1. Psychic determinism governs human behavior
    2. Unconscious processes occur in normal and abnormal mental functioning
    3. Repressed feelings associated with conflict—and their release—are the focus of the theory
    4. The topographic model of the mind includes the conscious, the preconscious, and the unconscious
    5. The structural model of the mind includes the id, the ego, and the superego
    6. Psychic energy derives from one's instincts or drives
    7. Everyone uses defense mechanisms
    8. Psychosexual development occurs in five stages
       a. Oral stage (0 to 18 months)
       b. Anal stage (18 months to age 3)

      c. Phallic stage (ages 3 to 5)

      d. Latency stage (age 5 to onset of puberty)

      e. Genital stage (pubescence to young adulthood)

C. Therapeutic process
   1. The therapist may use FREE ASSOCIATION, dream analysis, hypnosis, and interpretation to help the client recognize intrapsychic conflicts
   2. The client is motivated to work in therapy by TRANSFERENCE
   3. Psychoanalysis can involve up to five meetings a week for several years

D. Other psychoanalytic theorists
   1. Eric Erikson expanded psychosocial development to encompass the life cycle
   2. Anna Freud expanded the area of child psychology
   3. Melanie Klein developed play therapy in working with young children
   4. Karen Horney related behavior to cultural and interpersonal factors
   5. Freida Fromm-Reichman furthered the psychoanalytic theory of PSYCHOTIC BEHAVIOR
   6. Karl Menninger developed levels of psychic dysfunction

# VIII. Social model

A. General comments
   1. The social model is associated with Gerald Caplan and Thomas Szasz
   2. This model considers the impact of the social environment on an individual

B. Assumptions and key ideas
   1. The self emerges through social interaction
   2. Deviance is culturally defined; it is not an illness
   3. Society labels "undesirables" as mentally ill
   4. Diagnosis and institutionalization are used to exert social control over deviants
   5. An individual takes responsibility for behavior by deciding whether or not to conform to social expectations
   6. Social situations, such as poverty or inadequate education, can predispose an individual to mental illness
   7. Crises can trigger deviant behavior

C. Therapeutic process
   1. Therapy promotes freedom of choice and COMMUNITY MENTAL HEALTH
   2. The client defines the problem and initiates therapy
   3. The therapist (who may be professional or nonprofessional) collaborates with the client to promote change

## Points to remember

Assumptions about the development of personality and deviance vary by conceptual model.

The functions and roles of the therapist and the client differ within each conceptual model.

Using a holistic approach, nursing models consider the client's response to actual or potential health problems.

The nurse-client relationship is a collaboration, with the nurse acting as client advocate.

## Glossary

The following terms are defined in Appendix A, page 142.

| | |
|---|---|
| aversion therapy | operant conditioning |
| community mental health | psychosurgery |
| counter-conditioning | psychotic behavior |
| desensitization | rational-emotive therapy |
| encounter group therapy | reality therapy |
| existentialism | stressors |
| free association | token economy system |
| gestalt therapy | transference |
| holistic | transmethylation |
| neurotic behavior | |

## Study questions

To evaluate your understanding of this chapter, answer the following questions in the space provided; then compare your responses with the correct answers in Appendix B, page 149.

1. What key idea forms the basis of the behavioral model?

_____

2. What are the roles of the therapist and the client in the existential model?

_____

_____

3. What are the six phases of interpersonal development in the interpersonal model? _____

_____

4. In the medical model, how is the diagnosis recorded and classified? _____

_____

_____

5. What is the focus of nursing models? _____

_____

6. Who is the father of the psychoanalytic model? _____

_____

7. What are the roles of the client and the therapist in the social model?

_____

_____

## CHAPTER 2

# Roles and Functions of Psychiatric Nurses

## Learning objectives

Check off the following items once you've mastered them:

☐ Discuss how the role of psychiatric-mental health nursing has evolved, and describe its five components.

☐ List at least nine practice settings for psychiatric-mental health nurses.

☐ Identify at least seven roles and functions of psychiatric-mental health nurses.

☐ Name the six factors that determine the performance level of a psychiatric-mental health nurse.

# I. Historical trends in psychiatric nursing care

A. 1880 to 1914
   1. Provision of custodial care
   2. Attention to the client's physical needs
   3. Medication administration
   4. Assistance with hydrotherapy
   5. Encouragement of the client's participation in ward activities
   6. Kindness toward and tolerance of the client

B. 1915 to 1945
   1. Expansion of the nursing care role through SOMATIC THERAPIES (nurses expected to provide emotional and physical care)
   2. Recognition of the need for nurses with education and experience in psychiatry
   3. Integration of psychiatric nursing into generic nursing curricula

C. 1946 to 1962
   1. National Mental Health Act (1946), which authorized creation of the National Institute of Mental Health (NIMH) for research, training, and establishment of mental health centers
   2. Availability of federal funding for collegiate nursing education and graduate degrees
   3. Improvements in psychiatric nursing care standards
   4. Use of tranquilizers, which shifted the focus of nursing care to therapeutic relationships and contributed to the trend toward deinstitutionalization
   5. Development of psychiatric nursing theories as a basis for practice, including the work of Harry Stack Sullivan, whose theories helped define the nurse's role in MILIEU THERAPY
   6. Mental Health Survey Act (1955), which created the Joint Commission on Mental Illness and Health to evaluate the needs and resources of mentally ill persons in the United States
   7. Shift in treatment from institutions to community mental health centers, in accordance with the Report of the Joint Commission (1961)

D. 1963 to 1971
   1. Community Mental Health Act (1963), which encouraged graduate education for nurses
   2. Movement of psychiatric nurses into the community
   3. Expansion of the nurse's role to include promotion of mental health

E. 1972 to the present
   1. President's Commission on Mental Health (1978), which emphasized the need for more community-based services and for increased mental health funding
   2. Mental Health Systems Act (1980), which gave substance to the Commission's recommendations

3. Repeal of the Mental Health Systems Act (1981), cutting funds for psychological and social health services
4. Withdrawal of federal funding from nursing education and from clinical training in psychiatric-mental health nursing
5. Publication of revised Psychiatric and Mental Health Nursing Practice standards (1982)
6. Creation of a national center for nursing research at the National Institutes of Health (1985)
7. Creation of an NIMH task force on nursing (1987)
8. Establishment of the National Mental Health Leadership Forum (1989)

## II. Components of the psychiatric nursing role

A. An interpersonal process used to promote, maintain, restore, or rehabilitate an individual's mental health

B. A specialized area of nursing practice, as defined by the American Nurses' Association (ANA), that employs theories of human behavior as its science and "powerful use of self" as its art

C. A skill that draws on psychosocial and biophysical sciences and on theories of personality and human behavior

D. A profession that accepts individuals, families, groups, and communities as clients

E. A core mental health discipline, as recognized by the NIMH

## III. Practice settings

A. Psychiatric hospitals

B. Community mental health centers

C. General hospitals

D. Community health agencies

E. Outpatient clinics

F. Homes

G. Schools

H. Prisons

I. Health maintenance organizations

J. Private practices

K. Crisis units

L. Industrial centers

## IV. Current roles of psychiatric nurses

A. Staff nurses

B. Administrators

C. Consultants

D. Inservice educators

E. Clinical practitioners

F. Researchers

G. Program evaluators

H. Primary care providers

I. Liaisons between the client and other members of the health care delivery system

## V. Psychiatric nursing functions

A. General, as defined by the ANA
  1. Provide a therapeutic MILIEU
  2. Work to solve the client's current problems
  3. Fulfill a surrogate parent role
  4. Use somatic therapies to alleviate the client's health problems
  5. Educate consumers about factors (such as normal growth and development) that influence mental health
  6. Promote improved socioeconomic conditions
  7. Provide leadership to other personnel
  8. Conduct psychotherapy
  9. Engage in social and community mental health efforts

B. PRIMARY PREVENTION
  1. Conduct health education
  2. Improve socioeconomic conditions
  3. Offer consumer education about normal growth and development
  4. Provide referrals before symptoms develop
  5. Support family members
  6. Engage in community and political activity

C. SECONDARY PREVENTION
  1. Screen and evaluate clients promptly
  2. Visit the client at home
  3. Provide emergency treatment
  4. Provide a therapeutic milieu
  5. Supervise clients on medication
  6. Prevent suicide
  7. Counsel on a time-limited basis
  8. Provide CRISIS INTERVENTION

# A.N.A. STANDARDS OF PSYCHIATRIC AND MENTAL HEALTH NURSING PRACTICE

## PROFESSIONAL PRACTICE STANDARDS

### Standard 1. Theory
The nurse applies appropriate theory that is scientifically sound as a basis for decisions regarding nursing practice.

### Standard 2. Data Collection
The nurse continuously collects data that are comprehensive, accurate, and systematic.

### Standard 3. Diagnosis
The nurse utilizes nursing diagnoses and/or standard classification of mental disorders to express conclusions supported by recorded assessment data and current scientific premises.

### Standard 4. Planning
The nurse develops a nursing care plan with specific goals and interventions delineating nursing actions unique to each client's needs.

### Standard 5. Intervention
The nurse intervenes as guided by the nursing care plan to implement nursing actions that promote, maintain, or restore physical and mental health; prevent illness; and effect rehabilitation.

### Standard 5A. Intervention: Psychotherapeutic Interventions
The nurse uses psychotherapeutic interventions to assist clients in regaining or improving their previous coping abilities and to prevent further disability.

### Standard 5B. Intervention: Health Teaching
The nurse assists clients, families, and groups to achieve satisfying and productive patterns of living through health teaching.

### Standard 5C. Intervention: Activities of Daily Living
The nurse uses the activities of daily living in a goal-directed way to foster adequate self-care and physical and mental well-being of clients.

### Standard 5D. Intervention: Somatic Therapies
The nurse uses knowledge of somatic therapies and applies related clinical skills in working with clients.

### Standard 5E. Intervention: Therapeutic Environment
The nurse provides, structures, and maintains a therapeutic environment in collaboration with the client and other health care providers.

### Standard 5F. Intervention: Psychotherapy*
The nurse utilizes advanced clinical expertise in individual, group, and family psychotherapy; child psychotherapy; and other treatment modalities to function as a psychotherapist and recognizes professional accountability for nursing practice.

### Standard 6. Evaluation
The nurse evaluates client responses to nursing actions in order to revise the data base, nursing diagnoses, and nursing care plan.

## PROFESSIONAL PERFORMANCE STANDARDS

### Standard 7. Peer Review
The nurse participates in peer review and other means of evaluation to assure quality of nursing care provided for clients.

### Standard 8. Continuing Education
The nurse assumes responsibility for continuing education and professional development and contributes to the professional growth of others.

*(continued)*

*Specific to clinical specialists with a master's degree in psychiatric or mental health nursing

**A.N.A. STANDARDS OF PSYCHIATRIC AND MENTAL HEALTH NURSING PRACTICE** (continued)

**PROFESSIONAL PERFORMANCE STANDARDS** (continued)

**Standard 9. Interdisciplinary Collaboration**
The nurse collaborates with other health care providers in assessing, planning, implementing, and evaluating programs and other mental health activities.

**Standard 10. Utilization of Community Health Systems***
The nurse participates with other members of the community in assessing, planning, implementing, and evaluating mental health services and community systems that include the promotion of the broad continuum of primary, secondary, and tertiary prevention of mental illness.

**Standard 11. Research**
The nurse contributes to nursing and the mental health field through innovations in theory and practice and participation in research.

*Specific to clinical specialists with a master's degree in psychiatric or mental health nursing

From: *Standards of Psychiatric and Mental Health Nursing Practice*. Kansas City: American Nurses' Association, 1982. Used with permission.

   9.  Conduct psychotherapy
  10.  Initiate community and organizational interventions (for example, assisting with establishment of shelters for the homeless)

D. TERTIARY PREVENTION
  1.  Establish vocational training and rehabilitation programs
  2.  Establish aftercare programs
  3.  Recommend partial hospitalization, if appropriate

E. Indirect activities
  1.  Participate in inservice and continuing education
  2.  Pursue nursing administration
  3.  Supervise other personnel
  4.  Engage in consultation and research

## VI. Factors determining the performance level of psychiatric nurses

A. Nurse practice acts
  1.  Regulate entry into the profession and define the legal limits of nursing practice (all states)
  2.  Recognize the advanced practice of nurses (some states)

B. Education and experience
  1.  Generalists—licensed registered nurses directly involved in mental health and psychiatric nursing; must meet the profession's standards of knowledge, experience, and quality of care; baccalaureate in nursing required by 1998

    2. Specialists — have graduate education, supervised clinical experience, and depth of knowledge, competence, and skill in their practice

C. Certification
    1. Requires a formal review process by the ANA
    2. Provides credentials for clinical practice, which certifies the nurse as either a generalist or a specialist

D. Practice setting
    1. Organization's philosophy of mental illness, which helps shape the expectations of the client and the nurse
    2. Administrative policies, which either foster or limit full use of nursing services

E. Personal initiative
    1. Willingness to act as an agent of change
    2. Knowledge of one's strengths and weaknesses
    3. Realization of clinical competence

F. Professional standards
    1. Developed by the ANA in 1982
    2. Define practice and performance (see *ANA Standards of Psychiatric and Mental Health Nursing Practice*, page 13)

## Points to remember

Psychiatric nursing evolved in the late 19th and early 20th centuries.

Psychiatric nursing uses interpersonal processes to promote, maintain, or restore mental health.

Numerous practice settings are available to psychiatric nurses.

Psychiatric nursing includes both direct and indirect care.

Psychiatric nurses participate in primary, secondary, and tertiary levels of prevention.

## Glossary

The following terms are defined in Appendix A, page 142.

crisis intervention

secondary prevention

milieu

somatic therapies

milieu therapy

tertiary prevention

primary prevention

## Study questions

To evaluate your understanding of this chapter, answer the following questions in the space provided; then compare your responses with the correct answers in Appendix B, page 149.

1. What kinds of nursing care were delivered to mentally ill clients during the late 1800s and early 1900s? _____

    _____

2. What governmental legislation created the National Institute of Mental Health? _____

    _____

3. When did treatment for the mentally ill move from institutions to the community? _____

    _____

4. How does the American Nurses' Association define the psychiatric nursing role? _____

    _____

5. What are the psychiatric nursing functions in primary prevention? _____

    _____

6. How do psychiatric nurse generalists differ from psychiatric nurse specialists? _____

    _____

## CHAPTER 3

# Stress and Psychophysiologic Disorders

**Learning objectives**

Check off the following items once you've mastered them:

☐ Describe the four characteristics of stress.

☐ Discuss the four physiologic responses to stress.

☐ Name eight stress-related illnesses.

☐ Formulate nursing care goals and interventions for clients with stress-related illnesses.

## I. Characteristics of stress

A. Stress is a state of imbalance within an organism brought about by an actual or perceived disparity between environmental demands (STRESSORS) and the organism's capacity to cope with them

B. Stress manifests itself in various physiologic, emotional, and behavioral response patterns

C. Any emotion, activity, or situation that requires a response can produce stress

D. Three factors influence the stress response
   1. Intensity of the stimulus
   2. Duration of the stimulus
   3. Perception of control over the stimulus

## II. Adaptation: Physiologic responses to stress

A. General ADAPTATION syndrome (GAS)
   1. Alarm
   2. Resistance
   3. Exhaustion

B. Local adaptation syndrome
   1. Inflammatory, localized reaction to injury
   2. Reaction similar to GAS

C. FIGHT-OR-FLIGHT RESPONSE

D. Symptoms of stress
   1. Nervousness
   2. Inertia
   3. Insomnia
   4. Headache
   5. Dizziness
   6. Fainting
   7. Nightmares

## III. Stress-related illness

A. Characteristics
   1. Any experience perceived to be stressful may result in a psychophysiologic disorder
   2. Most clients do not consciously recognize stress
   3. Specific mind-body relationships are poorly understood by experts
   4. The primary behaviors observed are somatic symptoms

B. Theories about predisposing biological factors
   1. Endocrine activity affects personality
   2. Genetic factors have been proposed but not proved

      3. Target organs may be affected by specific stressors, but this theory is not supported by research

  C. Theories about psychological factors

      1. Many clinical experts contend that a relationship exists between personality type and specific psychophysiologic disorders

      2. Although specific psychological factors have been associated with certain physical conditions, no etiological theory has been proven

      3. The client's difficulty in dealing with feelings or in acknowledging their importance may contribute to a psychophysiologic disorder

  D. Psychophysiologic disorders

      1. Stress-related skin disorders may include allergy, eczema, hives, and acne

      2. Stress-related respiratory system disorders may include breathlessness, hyperventilation, hay fever, asthma, sinusitis, emphysema, and bronchial spasms

      3. Stress-related cardiovascular system disorders may include hypertension, migraine headaches, and coronary heart disease

      4. Stress-related endocrine system disorders may include diabetes mellitus, gonadal dysfunction, and adrenal dysfunction

      5. Stress-related musculoskeletal system disorders may include backaches and muscle cramps

      6. Stress-related gastrointestinal system disorders may include colitis, gastritis, constipation, obesity, hyperacidity, duodenal ulcer, and anorexia

      7. Stress-related genitourinary system disorders may include menstrual disturbances, impotence, and vaginismus

      8. In extreme cases, death may result (research suggests that this represents the exhaustion phase of GAS)

## IV. Nursing assessment data

  A. Complete physiologic assessment

  B. Thorough psychosocial assessment

  C. Measurement of stress level

  D. Investigation of coping abilities

  E. Identification of belief systems

  F. Examination of family dynamics

## V. Diagnoses

  A. Criteria

      1. Must reflect the complexity of the biopsychosocial interaction

      2. Must consider all aspects of the client's life that may be generating stress-related anxiety, as well as predisposing and precipitating stressors

      3. Must consider the client's stress level and coping skills

  B. Types of diagnoses

      1. *DSM-III-R* medical diagnoses: psychological factors affecting the physical condition (for example, conversion disorder or hypochondriasis)

      2. Primary NANDA diagnostic category: ineffective individual coping

## VI. General nursing care goals and interventions

  A. Maintain the client's biological integrity

  B. Offer support while establishing a trusting relationship

  C. Do not confront the client or attempt to explain unconscious psychodynamic processes to the client

  D. Teach the client to:

      1. Cope more effectively

      2. Experience feelings consciously and share feelings with others

      3. Reduce the frequency and intensity of existing stressors

      4. Modify stimuli that might generate further stress

  E. Show family members how to support the client's behavioral changes

  F. Refer the client and family to appropriate clinicians or agencies

## VII. Stress management strategies

  A. Progressive relaxation

  B. BIOFEEDBACK

  C. Meditation

  D. Hypnosis

  E. GUIDED IMAGERY

  F. Behavior modification

  G. Yoga

  H. Exercise and stretching

  I. ATTITUDINAL RESTRUCTURING

  J. AUTOGENIC TRAINING

  K. Stress DESENSITIZATION

  L. Massage

M. THERAPEUTIC TOUCH

N. Psychotherapy

O. Nutrition

P. Laughter

Q. Play

R. Music

## VIII. Evaluation

A. Base evaluation on identified client care goals

B. Do not interpret lack of goal achievement as failure

## Points to remember

Stress manifests itself in various physiologic, emotional, and behavioral response patterns.

General adaptation syndrome is a physiologic reaction to stress.

Health care providers must not ignore the psychological needs of clients with physical symptoms.

The nurse should offer support to clients with stress-related disorders.

Nursing interventions can enhance the client's ability to reduce and manage stress.

## Glossary

The following terms are defined in Appendix A, page 142.

| | |
|---|---|
| adaptation | fight-or-flight response |
| attitudinal restructuring | guided imagery |
| autogenic training | stressors |
| biofeedback | therapeutic touch |
| desensitization | |

## Study questions

To evaluate your understanding of this chapter, answer the following questions in the space provided; then compare your responses with the correct answers in Appendix B, page 150.

1. What is stress? _____

   _____

2. Which three factors influence the stress response? _____

   _____

3. What are the three phases of general adaptation syndrome? _____

   _____

4. Which two types of diagnoses are used to identify stress and psychobiologic

   disorders? _____

   _____

5. Which strategies can be used to manage stress? _____

   _____

## CHAPTER 4

# Dying and Grieving

**Learning objectives**

Check off the following items once you've mastered them:

☐ Identify at least five emotions common to dying clients.

☐ Describe nursing care goals and interventions for the dying client and family.

☐ Name at least three behaviors associated with uncomplicated, delayed, and distorted grief reactions.

☐ Identify four nursing care goals and interventions for clients experiencing uncomplicated grief reactions.

# I. Dying

A. Theoretical perspectives
  1. Natural death
     a. Occurs expectedly as a result of disease, thereby completing the life cycle
     b. Usually elicits an UNCOMPLICATED GRIEF REACTION from survivors because it is expected
  2. Sudden death
     a. Occurs without warning, thereby terminating the life cycle
     b. Usually elicits a more prolonged or complicated grief reaction from survivors because it is unexpected

B. Stages of coping with anticipated dying
  1. Denial
     a. Establishes a protective barrier
     b. Allows mobilization of other coping methods
     c. Should not be challenged by the nurse
     d. May manifest as an unwillingness to acknowledge symptoms, noncompliance, or refusal to discuss illness-related matters
  2. Anger
     a. Commonly occurs after the client perceives a loss of control
     b. Is usually directed toward others
  3. Bargaining
     a. Constitutes an attempt to postpone the inevitable
     b. Commonly involves the dying person making a secret pact with God
  4. Depression
  5. Acceptance
     a. Wishes to be left alone
     b. Becomes less involved with others
     c. Appears devoid of all feelings
     d. Experiences a sense of closure

C. Common emotions of clients anticipating death
  1. Loneliness
  2. Sorrow
  3. Fear of the unknown
  4. Fear of dying alone
  5. Loss of self-concept from altered body image
  6. Regression and dependence
  7. Loss of self-control
  8. Fear of suffering and pain

D. Nursing care goals for the client and family
  1. Assist the client in living more fully and comfortably until death
  2. Help the family support the client
  3. Encourage the client and family members to accept death

E. Nursing interventions for the client
   1. Maintain a secure, caring atmosphere
   2. Accept and support the client's denial as a necessary COPING MECHANISM
   3. Encourage the client to participate in decisions that affect the client's life
   4. Understand the client's anger
   5. Encourage the client to articulate needs and feelings
   6. Help the client schedule daily routines to include satisfying activities
   7. Assist the client in reviewing the past

F. Nursing interventions for the family
   1. Encourage the family to communicate openly with the client
   2. Recommend that family members help the client complete unfinished business (making a will; settling financial affairs)
   3. Reassure the client and family that anger, depression, guilt, and a sense of loss are normal stages of grieving
   4. Encourage family members to express their feelings about the client's anticipated death
   5. Help family members adapt to changes in roles or life-styles
   6. Enlist family members in caring for the client

G. Evaluation
   1. Note whether the client and family move toward acceptance of death
   2. Document evidence of maladaptive responses

## II. GRIEVING

A. Definitions
   1. Subjective response to the loss of a significant person or object
   2. Universal reaction that affects all aspects of one's life
   3. Emotion that typically impairs the ability to function
   4. Syndrome that usually has a predictable cause and effect

B. Symptoms
   1. Somatic distress
      a. Waves of distress lasting from 20 to 60 minutes
      b. Sighs and deep breathing when discussing grief
      c. Lack of strength
      d. Loss of appetite and sense of taste
      e. Tightness in throat
      f. Choking sensation accompanied by shortness of breath
   2. Preoccupation with image of the deceased person, characterized by:
      a. Daydreaming
      b. Mistaking others for the deceased person
      c. Becoming oblivious to surroundings
      d. Feeling a sense of unreality
      e. Fearing insanity

      3. Guilt
      4. Hostility
      5. Personality disorganization
         a. Loss of self-esteem
         b. Despair
         c. Transient hallucinations
         d. Overwhelming feelings of loneliness, fear, and helplessness

C. Types of grieving
    1. Uncomplicated grief reactions
      a. Shock and disbelief
      b. Heightened awareness
         (1) Intense and conflicting emotions, such as sadness and anger
         (2) Self-destructive behavior
         (3) Preoccupation with and yearning for the lost person
         (4) Guilt over perceived omissions
         (5) Acute symptoms of grief lasting 4 to 8 weeks
         (6) Disorganization of personality as hope of reunion is surrendered
      c. Reorganization, letting go, resolution
         (1) Detachment
         (2) Withdrawal
         (3) Investment of energy in new objects or people
         (4) Loss of future orientation
         (5) Painful review of memories
         (6) Process that typically lasts up to 1 year
    2. Delayed grief reaction
      a. Persistent absence of emotions
      b. Maladaptive response that can occur in any phase of the grieving process; anniversary day of loss may trigger underlying emotions
    3. Distorted grief reactions
      a. Excessive activity with no sense of loss
      b. Physical symptoms like those of the deceased person
      c. Psychophysiologic illness
      d. Progressive social isolation
      e. Extreme hostility
      f. Wooden and formal conduct
      g. Clinical depression
      h. Activities detrimental to one's social and economic good
      i. Euphoria

D. Nursing care goals and interventions
    1. For uncomplicated grief reactions
      a. Understand personal feelings about and reactions to loss
      b. Support a dying client who is grieving
         (1) Establish rapport and build trust

(2) Provide ANTICIPATORY GUIDANCE by helping the client prepare for death and its consequences for the client's family

(3) Encourage the client to express feelings candidly

(4) Discourage the client from lingering in one stage of grieving or from using activities to avoid grieving

(5) Provide the client with opportunities to release tension and guilt

(6) Promote an adequate balance of rest, sleep, and activity

(7) Avoid use of daytime sedatives and tranquilizers

(8) Discourage dependence on staff members or others

(9) Encourage the client to interact with others and to plan for the future

(10) Mobilize the client's support systems

   c. Support the family

      (1) Communicate news of the client's death to the family as a group, in a private setting

      (2) Respect their religious and cultural beliefs and practices

      (3) Permit outward expression of grief

      (4) Listen attentively, and express sympathy

2. For delayed grief reaction

   a. Help the client identify underlying emotions associated with the loss

   b. Help the client progress through the stages of normal grieving

3. For distorted grief reactions

   a. Set goals according to the client's needs (for instance, promoting independence in a client who has become overly dependent)

   b. Direct interventions toward specific behaviors (for instance, focusing on personal hygiene if a client's withdrawn behavior leads the client to neglect hygiene needs)

E. Evaluation

1. Note the client's progression through the stages of grieving

2. Document evidence of or changes in maladaptive emotional responses

## Points to remember

The nurse should not challenge denial as an initial coping mechanism.

Grief is a universal response to loss.

Uncomplicated grief reaction usually lasts about 1 year.

The anniversary of a loss may trigger a delayed grief reaction.

General nursing care goals for uncomplicated grief reactions should support the grieving process.

## Glossary

The following terms are defined in Appendix A, page 142.

anticipatory guidance

coping mechanism

grieving

uncomplicated grief reaction

## Study questions

To evaluate your understanding of this chapter, answer the following questions in the space provided; then compare your responses with the correct answers in Appendix B, page 150.

1. What are the five stages of coping with anticipated dying? _____

_____

2. What is the focus of nursing care goals for the dying client and family?

_____

_____

3. What are the three phases of uncomplicated grief? _____ _____

_____

4. Which symptoms are important in evaluating a grieving client? _____

_____

_____

5. How should a nurse manage a client who is experiencing a distorted grief

   reaction? _____

_____

## CHAPTER 5

# Alterations in Self-Concept

## Learning objectives

Check off the following items once you've mastered them:

☐ Identify five stressors that affect self-concept.

☐ Describe three behaviors associated with alterations in self-concept.

☐ Formulate individualized nursing diagnoses for clients experiencing alterations in self-concept.

☐ Develop a nursing care plan, including goals and interventions, for meeting the needs of clients experiencing alterations in self-concept.

# I. Self-concept

A. Definitions
  1. All notions, beliefs, and convictions that constitute a person's self-knowledge and that, if positive, allow an individual to function more effectively
  2. A determinant of a person's relationships with others
  3. A frame of reference by which each person interacts with the world
  4. The consequence, in part, of experiences with significant others

B. Components
  1. BODY IMAGE
     a. Attitude toward one's body, which usually mirrors self-concept
     b. Sum of conscious and unconscious attitudes, continually modified by one's perceptions and experiences
     c. Significant influence on self-esteem and role perception
  2. IDENTITY
     a. Awareness of oneself
     b. Consequence of self-observation and judgment
     c. Synthesis of self-representations into an organized whole
     d. Consciousness of oneself as an individual
     e. Concept that emerges in adolescence
     f. Ego identity
        (1) Recognition of the self as separate from others
        (2) Acceptance of one's sexuality
        (3) Compatibility among other aspects of self
        (4) Congruence between self-regard and societal regard
        (5) Awareness of relationships among past, present, and future
        (6) Realistic self-goals
     g. Object of maturational, cultural, and physiologic stressors
  3. Roles
     a. Consist of socially expected behavior associated with one's function within the societal group
     b. Provide a way to test identity
     c. Enhance self-esteem when they are congruent with self-ideals
     d. Lead to role disturbances when conflicts emerge between independent and dependent functioning
     e. Produce role strain from stress associated with role expectations
     f. Lead to role conflict when a person is subjected to simultaneous contradictory expectations or when an individual's or society's expectations of role behavior are incongruent
     g. Can result in role ambiguity when knowledge about specific role expectations is limited
     h. May produce role overload when the individual is faced with an overly complex set of roles
  4. SELF-ESTEEM
     a. Individual's sense of self-worth

      b. Beliefs that originate in childhood and that are modified throughout life

      c. Internalization of the reactions of others; anxiety occurs when the self is threatened

      d. High self-esteem: prerequisite to SELF-ACTUALIZATION

      e. Low self-esteem: factor in poorly developed interpersonal relationships

   5. Self-ideals

      a. Individual's perception of how to behave, based on personal standards and societal norms

      b. Standards influenced by abilities, cultural factors, ambitions, desire to succeed and avoid failure, anxiety, and inferiority

      c. Prerequisite for mental health: congruency between self-ideals and self-concept

## II. Characteristics of a healthy personality

A. Positive and accurate body image

B. Realistic self-ideal

C. Positive self-concept

D. High self-esteem

E. Clear sense of identity

F. Openness to others

## III. Behaviors associated with altered self-concept

A. Low self-esteem
1. Self-derision and criticism
2. Minimization of one's ability
3. Guilt and worry
4. Physical manifestations (such as substance abuse or psychosomatic illness)
5. Ambivalence or procrastination
6. Denial of pleasure to oneself
7. Disturbed interpersonal relationships
8. Withdrawal from reality
9. Destructive behavior (toward self or others)

B. Identity confusion
1. Lack of sense of continuity between past and present
2. High degree of anxiety
3. Fluctuations in feelings about self
4. Uncertainty about self-characteristics
5. Withdrawal from reality
6. Exaggerated sense of self-importance

C. Depersonalization
   1.  Inability to distinguish between internal and external stimuli
   2.  Difficulty distinguishing self from others
   3.  Feelings that the body has an unreal quality
   4.  Estrangement
   5.  Confusion about sexuality
   6.  Absence of emotion
   7.  Loss of spontaneity
   8.  Withdrawal
   9.  Disturbed perceptions of time and space
   10. Impaired judgment and thinking
   11. Loss of impulse control
   12. Inability to derive sense of accomplishment

## IV. Diagnosis

A. *DSM-III-R* medical diagnoses
   1.  Multiple personality
   2.  Psychogenic fugue
   3.  Psychogenic amnesia
   4.  Depersonalization disorder
   5.  Dissociative disorder
   6.  Narcissistic personality disorder
   7.  Borderline personality disorder
   8.  Anorexia nervosa
   9.  Bulimia nervosa

B. Primary NANDA diagnostic categories
   1.  Body image disturbance
   2.  Self-esteem disturbance
   3.  Altered role performance
   4.  Personality identity disturbance

## V. Nursing care goals and interventions

A. General comments
   1.  Ensure the client's active participation in planning and implementation of treatment
   2.  Assess the client's readiness for growth
   3.  Establish clear and explicit goals
   4.  Emphasize strengths rather than the pathologic condition
   5.  Use problem-solving techniques
   6.  Focus on the present

B. Primary goals
   1.  Increase the client's self-realization and self-acceptance
   2.  Help the client demonstrate increased confidence and self-worth

C. Interventions to expand the client's SELF-AWARENESS
   1. Accept the client unconditionally
   2. Listen attentively
   3. Encourage the client to discuss thoughts and feelings
   4. Respond nonjudgmentally
   5. Convey the expectation that the client is capable of self-help
   6. Identify the client's ego strengths
   7. Confirm the client's identity
   8. Reduce the client's anxiety level
   9. Set limits on appropriate behavior
   10. Assist with personal hygiene
   11. Provide activities that can be easily accomplished
   12. Increase the number and complexity of activities gradually

D. Interventions to encourage self-exploration
   1. Help the client accept positive and negative thoughts and emotions
   2. Help the client identify strengths, weaknesses, and self-criticisms
   3. Have the client describe a self-ideal
   4. Help the client describe how he or she relates to others
   5. Respond with empathy
   6. Teach the client to recognize conflict and maladaptive coping

E. Interventions to foster self-evaluation
   1. Help identify relevant stressors, unrealistic goals, faulty perceptions, strengths, and maladaptive responses
   2. Explore coping resources
   3. Use such techniques as SUPPORTIVE CONFRONTATION, ROLE CLARIFICATION, and PSYCHODRAMA

F. Interventions to help formulate a realistic plan of action
   1. Mutually identify adaptive coping responses
   2. Encourage the client to formulate self-goals and to try new behaviors
   3. Discuss the consequences of each goal
   4. Use such techniques as ROLE REVERSAL, ROLE MODELING, ROLE PLAYING, and VISUALIZATION

G. Interventions to assist in goal achievement
   1. Provide opportunities to experience success
   2. Reinforce healthy aspects of the client's coping skills
   3. Help identify and obtain needed resources
   4. Organize group activities
   5. Allow time to change
   6. Provide support and positive reinforcement

## VI. Evaluation

A. Note the client's ability to identify stressors

B. Document use of adaptive coping responses

## Points to remember

A healthy personality is characterized by a positive and accurate body image, realistic ideals, a positive self-concept, high self-esteem, a clear sense of identity, and openness toward others.

Behaviors associated with altered self-concept are varied but usually reflect low self-esteem, identity confusion, depersonalization, disturbed body image, and negative or delinquent identity.

The client must actively participate in treatment.

Nursing interventions must focus on assisting the client in problem solving.

## Glossary

The following terms are defined in Appendix A, page 142.

| | |
|---|---|
| body image | role reversal |
| identity | self-actualization |
| psychodrama | self-awareness |
| role clarification | self-esteem |
| role modeling | supportive confrontation |
| role playing | visualization |

## Study questions

To evaluate your understanding of this chapter, answer the following questions in the space provided; then compare your responses with the correct answers in Appendix B, pages 150 and 151.

1. What are the five components of self-concept? _____

   _____

2. What are the three categories of behavior associated with an altered self-concept? _____

   _____

3. What are the primary goals of the nurse when dealing with a client who is experiencing an alteration in self-concept? _____

   _____

4. How can the nurse intervene to assist the client with self-evaluation?

   _____

   _____

## CHAPTER 6

# Anxiety

## Learning objectives

Check off the following items once you've mastered them:

☐ Name the seven characteristics of anxiety.

☐ Discuss five theories on the origin of anxiety.

☐ Describe physiologic, behavioral, cognitive, and affective responses to anxiety.

☐ Develop nursing care goals and interventions for a client with anxiety.

## I. Characteristics

A. Consequence of and behavioral response to stress, changes, or threats to one's SELF-CONCEPT

B. Uneasiness caused by conflicts and frustrations that tax one's coping skills

C. State of unexplained discomfort

D. Source of energy that can be used constructively or destructively

E. Nonspecific feeling of dread accompanied by symptoms of physiologic stress

## II. Theories on the origin of anxiety

A. Psychoanalytic view (Freud)
1. Primary anxiety, a state of trauma and tension first produced by external causes, originates during birth
2. Subsequent anxiety is the emotional conflict between the primitive impulses of the ID and the regulatory function of the SUPEREGO

B. Interpersonal view (Sullivan)
1. Anxiety originates in the early bond between mother and child
2. The condition is related to fear of disapproval
3. Developmental trauma leads to specific vulnerabilities and anxiety
4. In later life, anxiety arises when the person perceives unfavorable responses from others
5. Anger commonly results from a mild or moderate level of anxiety

C. Behavioral views
1. Anxiety is a product of frustration generated when desired goals are not attained
2. No single theorist is associated with behavioral views on anxiety

D. Learning views
1. A learned drive, such as anxiety, is based on an innate desire to avoid pain
2. Individuals exposed in early life to intense fears are more likely to experience anxiety

E. Conflict view
1. Anxiety arises when one must choose between two opposing drives or interests
2. No single theorist is associated with the conflict view on anxiety

## III. Precipitating stressors

A. May be positive or negative

B. Can have physiologic, psychological, or environmental origins

C. May be perceived subjectively

    D. Can arise from threats to biological integrity

    E. Can arise from threats to self-esteem
        1. Unmet expectations
        2. Unfulfilled needs for status and prestige
        3. Anticipated disapproval
        4. Inability to gain recognition from others
        5. Guilt

## IV. Levels of anxiety

    A. Mild
        1. Heightens alertness
        2. Widens perceptual field
        3. Enhances learning

    B. Moderate
        1. Limits one's focus to immediate concerns
        2. Narrows perceptual field
        3. Produces selective inattention

    C. Severe
        1. Greatly reduces perceptual field
        2. Focuses one's attention on details of immediate concern
        3. Directs behavior toward getting relief
        4. Requires the person to seek guidance from others to focus on other areas

    D. Panic
        1. Distorts perceptions
        2. Severely impairs rational thought
        3. Diminishes ability to focus, even with direction from others
        4. Increases motor activity
        5. Decreases ability to relate to others

## V. Physiologic responses to anxiety

    A. Cardiovascular
        1. Palpitations
        2. Tachycardia
        3. Increased or decreased blood pressure
        4. Faintness

    B. Respiratory
        1. Rapid, shallow breathing
        2. Shortness of breath or gasping
        3. Chest pressure
        4. Lump in the throat or choking sensation

   C. Neuromuscular
      1. Increased reflexes
      2. Eyelid twitching
      3. Insomnia
      4. Fidgeting or pacing
      5. Generalized weakness

   D. Gastrointestinal
      1. Loss of appetite or revulsion toward food
      2. Abdominal discomfort or pain
      3. Nausea
      4. Heartburn
      5. Diarrhea

   E. Genitourinary
      1. Sudden urge to urinate
      2. Frequent urination

   F. Integumentary
      1. Flushing or pallor
      2. Sweating
      3. Itching
      4. Hot and cold spells

## VI. Behavioral responses to anxiety

   A. Restlessness

   B. Physical tension

   C. Tremors

   D. Startle reaction

   E. Rapid speech

   F. Lack of coordination

   G. Interpersonal withdrawal

   H. Avoidance

   I. Hyperventilation

## VII. Cognitive responses to anxiety

   A. Impaired attention

   B. Inadequate concentration

   C. Preoccupation

   D. Forgetfulness

   E. Blocking of thoughts

F. Confusion

G. Loss of objectivity

H. Fear

## VIII. Affective responses to anxiety

A. Edginess

B. Impatience

C. Uneasiness and tension

D. Fear

E. Jumpiness

## IX. Coping strategies

A. Task-oriented
1. Attack behavior: may be destructive if aggressive or constructive if self-assertive
2. Physical or emotional withdrawal: may be destructive if it results in isolation
3. Compromise: usually constructive

B. Ego-oriented
1. Unconscious defense mechanisms (such as denial or intellectualization) used to protect self when task-oriented strategies are unsuccessful
2. Can be detrimental and result in ego disintegration if used to an extreme

## X. Identifying nursing problems

A. Identify the client's anxiety level and its overall effect

B. Determine whether the client's DEFENSE MECHANISMS are constructive or destructive

## XI. Primary NANDA diagnostic categories

A. Anxiety

B. Ineffective individual coping

C. Fear

## XII. Nursing care goals

A. Increase the client's ability to tolerate mild anxiety, and show how to use that ability consciously and constructively

B. Aid the client in problem solving

C. Provide a safe, secure environment

D. Promote the client's self-esteem

## XIII. Nursing interventions

A. For moderate anxiety levels
1. Help the client recognize anxiety and underlying feelings
2. Design an individualized teaching plan to increase the client's knowledge of stressors, coping mechanisms, and responses to anxiety
3. Explore alternate coping strategies
4. Promote relaxation

B. For severe and panic anxiety levels
1. Stay with the client
2. Remain calm, and try to reduce the client's anxiety
3. Reduce stimuli
4. Use short, simple sentences
5. Assess personal anxiety level
6. Administer medications, as needed
7. Help channel the client's energy constructively
8. Encourage the client to eat nutritious foods
9. Suggest activities to promote sleep at bedtime

## XIV. Evaluation

A. Periodically judge the adequacy, effectiveness, appropriateness, efficiency, and flexibility of nursing goals and actions

B. Regularly evaluate personal strengths, limitations, and anxiety level

## Points to remember

Anxiety is sometimes experienced as unexplained discomfort.

Precipitating stressors include threats to biological integrity and to self-esteem.

Individuals exhibit physiologic, behavioral, cognitive, and affective responses to anxiety.

Mild anxiety enhances learning.

The overall goal of nursing intervention is to help the client develop the capacity to tolerate moderate anxiety and use it consciously and constructively.

## Glossary

The following terms are defined in Appendix A, page 142.

defense mechanisms

id

self-concept

superego

## Study questions

To evaluate your understanding of this chapter, answer the following questions in the space provided; then compare your responses to the correct answers in Appendix B, page 151.

1. How does Freud describe anxiety? _____

   _____

2. What are the three effects of moderate anxiety? _____

   _____

3. Which physiologic responses of the cardiovascular system would be important to assess during an examination of an anxious client? _____

   _____

4. What are the six affective responses to anxiety? _____

   _____

5. What is the most important nursing intervention for dealing with a client experiencing panic? _____

   _____

## CHAPTER 7

# Disordered Behaviors Associated with Anxiety

## Learning objectives

Check off the following items once you've mastered them:

☐ Identify at least eight characteristics of disturbed coping patterns seen in disordered behaviors associated with anxiety.

☐ Discuss several characteristic behaviors associated with each of the anxiety disorders, somatoform disorders, and dissociative disorders.

☐ Name five general nursing care goals for clients experiencing disordered behaviors associated with anxiety.

☐ Formulate intervention strategies for clients with anxiety disorders, somatoform disorders, or dissociative disorders.

## I. General characteristics of disturbed coping patterns

A. Inability to make choices

B. Internal conflict beyond conscious control

C. Repetition of thoughts and actions

D. State of sustained imbalance

E. ALIENATION or a feeling that thoughts and feelings are unrelated

F. Stress caused by EGO-DYSTONIC BEHAVIORS

G. Secondary gain (for example, getting increased attention from others as a result of being ill)

H. Manifestations of ritualistic, avoidant, clinging, distancing, and overly dramatic behaviors

I. Somatic symptoms that have no physical basis

J. Episodic amnesia

K. Multiple personalities

L. Underlying anxiety

## II. Anxiety disorder: Generalized anxiety state

A. Characteristics
1. Generalized, persistent anxiety; usually only mildly incapacitating
2. Symptoms unrelated to any other mental disorder; can persist for 1 month
3. Minimum client age for diagnosis: 18 years; median age at onset: 25 years
4. Depression as a major disabling side effect
5. Possible suicide attempts

B. Signs and symptoms
1. Motor tension: fidgeting, easy startle reflex, muscle twitching, trembling, strained expression, fatigue, inability to relax
2. Autonomic hyperactivity: sweating, flushing or pallor, elevated pulse and respiration rate, cold or clammy hands, diarrhea, frequent urination, pounding heart, upset stomach, light-headedness, dizziness, hot or cold spells, tingling of hands or feet
3. Apprehension: worry, anxiety, repetitive thoughts, fears of grave misfortune or death
4. Vigilance and scanning: overattention to surroundings, hypersensitivity, distractibility, inability to concentrate, impatience, irritability

C. Nursing interventions
   1. Observe for signs of mounting anxiety, and take direct measures to moderate it
   2. Teach the client to detect anxiety by making thoughtful observations
   3. Do not validate or encourage the client's use of destructive coping mechanisms
   4. Discuss options for meeting the client's needs
   5. Negotiate a contract to work on goals
   6. Alter the environment to reduce the anxiety or to meet the client's needs

## III. Anxiety disorder: Phobias

A. Characteristics
   1. Intense, irrational fear of an external object, activity, or situation
   2. Fear that persists even though the client recognizes its irrationality
   3. Tendency toward drug and alcohol abuse
   4. Resistance to insight-oriented therapies

B. Signs and symptoms
   1. Persistent fear of specific places or things
   2. Displacement and SYMBOLIZATION
   3. Disruption in social or work life
   4. Panic when confronted by the feared object

C. Nursing interventions
   1. Assist in desensitizing the client
   2. Demonstrate progressive relaxation techniques
   3. Suggest that the client substitute an alternate behavior
   4. Demonstrate healthier ways of coping

## IV. Anxiety disorder: Obsessive-compulsive disorder

A. Characteristics
   1. Acute attacks, commonly triggered by stressful incidents
   2. Behaviors substituted for relating to others
   3. Distress

B. Signs and symptoms
   1. Repetitive thoughts that the client cannot control or exclude from consciousness
   2. Recurring, irresistible impulses to perform an action
   3. Defense mechanisms, such as isolation, UNDOING, REACTION FORMATION, and MAGICAL THINKING

C. Nursing interventions
   1. Do not set direct limits
   2. Carefully weigh any interference with compulsive rituals
   3. Maintain a calm environment

    4. Remain sympathetic
    5. Avoid judging the client
    6. Make reasonable requests for the client to change
    7. Explain the reasons for change
    8. Engage in a constructive activity
    9. Reinforce nonritualistic behavior while encouraging the client's efforts to explore the meaning and purpose of behaviors
   10. Allow time for calming rituals (such as pacing) to show their effectiveness in reducing anxiety
   11. Desensitize the client toward feared objects or situations
   12. Teach relaxation techniques

## V. Anxiety disorder: Post-traumatic stress disorder

A. Characteristics
    1. Stressors related to actual experiences; usually traceable to a traumatic event
    2. Acute, chronic, or delayed reactions

B. Signs and symptoms
    1. Flashbacks
    2. Dreams
    3. Nightmares
    4. Detachment
    5. Emotional numbness

C. Nursing interventions
    1. Encourage the client to explore the meaning of the event
    2. Assist the client with problem solving

## VI. SOMATOFORM DISORDERS, CONVERSION DISORDERS, PSYCHOGENIC PAIN, and HYPOCHONDRIASIS

A. Characteristics
    1. Symptoms that carry a symbolic meaning
    2. Frequent remissions and exacerbations

B. Signs and symptoms
    1. Physical symptoms without evidence of organic cause
    2. Absence of psychological symptoms
    3. Inability to resist distraction

C. Nursing interventions
    1. Rule out any organic problems
    2. Be aware of personal responses to the client
    3. Remember that the client does not intentionally produce symptoms
    4. Avoid reinforcing the symptoms
    5. Assess the symbolic meaning of symptoms
    6. Encourage the client to express underlying anxiety

7. Increase the client's self-esteem
8. Set limits for the client

## VII. Dissociative disorders: Psychogenic amnesia, PSYCHOGENIC FUGUE, multiple personality, DEPERSONALIZATION disorder

A. Characteristics
   1. Triggerd by severe psychosocial stress
   2. Manifested by repression of or dissociation from anxiety-laden experiences, conflicts, aspects of self, or traumatic experiences
   3. Shown by separation of portions of ego from total personality

B. Signs and symptoms
   1. Denial
   2. Ego-splitting
   3. Alteration of mental functions
   4. Preoccupation with somatic symptoms
   5. Amnesia
   6. Multiple personalities

C. Nursing interventions
   1. Promote the client's self-actualization
   2. Encourage greater self-understanding
   3. Assess readiness for growth
   4. Identify realistic short-term goals
   5. Encourage exploration of feelings
   6. Focus on the client, not on symptoms

## VIII. General nursing care goals for disordered behaviors associated with anxiety

A. Encourage the client to express anxious feelings as they occur

B. Encourage the client to identify methods of coping with anxiety without avoidance or ritualistic or somatic behavior

C. Help the client identify feelings as well as realistic strengths and weaknesses

D. Encourage the client to describe how he or she contributes to the behavior pattern

E. Aid the client in evaluating relationships realistically

F. Teach the client to exercise self-control

G. Show the client ways of meeting personal needs

## IX. Intervention strategies

A. Psychopharmacology (antianxiety medications)

B. Individual psychotherapy

C. Behavior modification

D. Group therapy

## X. Evaluation

A. Use identified client care goals as a basis for evaluation

B. Identify reasons for nonachievement of goals

C. List outcomes expected by the nurse and the client

## Points to remember

Clients who experience disordered behaviors associated with anxiety exhibit specific disturbed coping patterns.

The goals for nursing intervention in such cases must be realistic.

The nurse must monitor personal anxiety level.

Clients who experience disturbed coping patterns associated with anxiety perceive distress but cannot successfully alter their behavior.

Nursing care goals should include helping the client learn how to cope with anxiety-laden experiences.

## Glossary

The following terms are defined in Appendix A, page 142.

| | |
|---|---|
| alienation | psychogenic fugue |
| conversion disorder | psychogenic pain |
| depersonalization | reaction formation |
| ego-dystonic behaviors | somatoform disorders |
| hypochondriasis | symbolization |
| magical thinking | undoing |

## Study questions

To evaluate your understanding of this chapter, answer the following questions in the space provided; then compare your responses with the correct answers in Appendix B, page 151.

1. What is the minimum age for a client to be diagnosed with generalized anxiety state? _____

_____

2. What the key sign of a client with a phobia? _____

_____

3. What are the key signs and symptoms a nurse will notice when assessing a client with an obsessive-compulsive disorder? _____

_____

4. How should a nurse intervene when dealing with a client experiencing a post-traumatic stress disorder? _____

_____

5. What is the focus of nursing interventions for a client with a dissociative disorder? _____

_____

6. What are the four intervention strategies for a client with an anxiety disorder? _____

_____

## CHAPTER 8

# Mood Disorders

## Learning objectives

Check off the following items once you've mastered them:

☐ Discuss six etiological theories of mood disorders.

☐ Identify four special treatment measures for mood disorders.

☐ Explain the primary behavioral characteristics of depressive and manic disorders.

☐ List at least six nursing diagnoses appropriate for clients who experience mood disorders.

☐ Describe nursing care goals and strategies for intervening with clients who experience mood disorders.

# I. Introduction

A. A mood disorder is a severe disturbance in AFFECT manifested by extreme sadness or euphoria

B. Degrees of severity and duration vary

C. Maladaptive behavior may develop after a personal loss

# II. Classification

A. Etiology
  1. Exogenous: the result of external loss or event
  2. Endogenous: without apparent external cause

B. Symptomatology
  1. Reactive: a reaction to bereavement
  2. Endogenous: without apparent external cause

C. Activity
  1. Retarded
  2. Agitated

D. Mood changes
  1. Unipolar: only episodes of DEPRESSION
  2. Bipolar: MANIA alternating with depression

E. *DSM-III-R* medical diagnoses
  1. Bipolar disorders, including manic and depressive disorders and cyclothymia
  2. Depressive disorders, including major depression and dysthymia

# III. Etiology

A. Genetic
  1. Mode of genetic transmission remains controversial
  2. Studies using genetic markers suggest that bipolar disorder is transmitted by the X-linked dominant gene
  3. Incidence is greater in relatives than in the general population
  4. The concordance rate is greater in monozygotic than in dizygotic twins
  5. Onset may occur without a precipitating stressor

B. Biological
  1. Biogenic amine hypothesis: excessive or insufficient availability of one or more neurotransmitters in the brain
  2. Electrolyte metabolism: disturbance in the distribution of sodium and potassium across cell membranes
  3. Neuroendocrine abnormalities: abnormal levels of cortisol, human growth hormone, and thyroid stimulating hormone
  4. Catecholamine deficiency or excess in the central nervous system

5. Biological rhythm disturbance
6. Treatment: pharmacologic therapy

C. Aggression-turned-inward theory (Sigmund Freud)
   1. Aggression accompanied by feelings of guilt
   2. Inability to express anger outwardly
   3. Validation of emotions unavailable empirically
   4. Treatment: expressing anger outwardly

D. Object-loss theory (J. Bowlby, R. Spitz, J. Robertson)
   1. Traumatic separation from significant persons or objects early in life
   2. Connection between early loss and adult depression unproven
   3. Treatment: coming to terms with early loss

E. Cognitive model (Aaron Beck)
   1. Depression resulting from negative view of self
   2. Negative cognitive set
   3. View of adverse event as a personal shortcoming; expectations of failure
   4. Depression developing over weeks
   5. Model supported by clinical and experimental studies
   6. Treatment: changing the thought process

F. Learned helplessness (Martin Seligman)
   1. Belief that no one will help and that one has no control over what happens
   2. Definition applies to a behavioral state and a personality trait
   3. Negative expectations lead to hopelessness, passivity, and nonassertiveness
   4. Syndrome cannot be empirically validated
   5. Treatment: regaining control

G. Behavioral model (P. Lewinsohn)
   1. Depression caused by person-behavior-environment interaction
   2. Low rate of positive reinforcement or lack of rewarding interactions preceding depression
   3. Treatment: increasing positively reinforcing interactions

H. Sociological theories and stress factors
   1. Loss
   2. Major life events
   3. Role strain
   4. Change in familiar environment
   5. Change in economic conditions or coping resources
   6. Physiologic changes
   7. Theory supported by research findings

# IV. Epidemiology

A. Mood disorders constitute the most common psychiatric disorder

B. Study is impeded by problems of definition and diagnosis

C. Mood disorders are responsible for 75% of psychiatric hospitalizations

D. Major depression is twice as common among women as among men

E. Onset of unipolar disorder occurs in the mid- to late-thirties; bipolar disorders, in the late twenties

## V. Special treatment measures

A. Electroconvulsive therapy (ECT)
 1. This therapy requires complete medical evaluation
 2. The client must not eat or drink after midnight before therapy
 3. A nurse must remove the client's shoes or slippers and any dentures or metal hairpins
 4. An anesthesiologist administers a short-acting anesthetic and inserts an artificial airway before the electric charge
 5. The client's arms should be restrained at the side
 6. Several electrodes are placed on the client's temples
 7. The electric current produces a tonic seizure lasting 5 to 15 seconds and a clonic seizure lasting 10 to 60 seconds
 8. A course of therapy entails three treatments a week on alternate days
 9. The client will experience confusion and forgetfulness, which usually disappear with time
 10. After treatment, the nurse should reorient the client and record vital signs every 15 minutes

B. Antidepressant medication
 1. Monoamine oxidase inhibitors
 2. Tricyclic antidepressants
 3. Amoxapine
 4. Maprotiline
 5. Second-generation antidepressants
 6. Nontricyclic drugs

C. Lithium therapy for bipolar disorders; carbamazepine as an alternative

D. Group and individual therapies
 1. Not effective when used alone
 2. Useful sometimes when combined with psychopharmacologic therapy

E. Phototherapy

F. Sleep manipulation

## VI. Primary NANDA diagnostic categories

A. Anxiety

B. Impaired verbal communication

C. Ineffective individual coping

D. Dysfunctional grieving

E. Hopelessness

F. Potential for injury

G. Altered nutrition (less than body requirements)

H. Powerlessness

I. Self-care deficit

J. Self-esteem disturbance

K. Sexual dysfunction

L. Sleep pattern disturbance

M. Social isolation

N. Spiritual distress

O. Altered thought processes

P. Potential for self-directed violence

## VII. Depressive reactions

A. Assessment: Characteristics of mild depression
   1. Transitory experience
   2. Condition commonly triggered by life events
   3. Part of normal grieving
   4. Manifestations: almost always emotions (for instance, sadness)
   5. Physiologic changes: alterations in sleep patterns
   6. Cognitive changes: decreased alertness, difficulty thinking logically, difficulty concentrating
   7. Behavioral changes: crying, withdrawal, irritability, increased use of alcohol or drugs

B. Assessment: Characteristics of moderate depression
   1. Depression that persists over time
   2. Condition that forces the client to seek help
   3. Affective changes: despondency, dejection, gloom, low self-esteem, powerlessness, helplessness, inability to experience pleasure
   4. Cognitive changes: slow thinking, narrowing of interests, indecisiveness, self-doubt, rumination, pessimism
   5. Potential for suicide attempt
   6. Behavioral changes: withdrawal, tears, irritability, poor hygiene, slow movement and speech, agitation, increased use of alcohol or drugs
   7. Physiologic changes: somatic complaints, anorexia, weight loss, fatigue, sleep disturbance

C. Assessment: Characteristics of severe depression
   1. Intense, pervasive, and persistent depression
   2. Altered reality orientation
   3. Affective changes: despair and hopelessness, worthlessness, guilt, valuelessness, loneliness
   4. Cognitive changes: confusion, indecisiveness, inability to concentrate, lack of motivation, intense self-blame and self-deprecation, wish to die, possible delusions or hallucinations
   5. Behavioral changes: psychomotor retardation or aimless agitation, poor posture, decreased speech, slow responses, unkempt appearance, social withdrawal
   6. Physiologic changes: constipation, urine retention, amenorrhea, lack of sexual interest, impotence, marked weight loss, insomnia

D. Nursing care goals
   1. Promote adequate nutrition, hydration, elimination, rest, sleep, and activity
   2. Stop withdrawn behavior
   3. Prevent the client from self-harm
   4. Decrease disorientation, ruminations, hallucinations, and delusions
   5. Promote feelings of self-worth and articulation of feelings

E. Nursing interventions: Physical needs
   1. Monitor and record nutritional intake
   2. Weigh the client daily
   3. Encourage small, frequent high-fiber meals and foods easily chewed; stay with the client during meals
   4. Teach methods to help the client relax and sleep
   5. Assist the client in getting out of bed and taking care of personal hygiene while encouraging the client to initiate self-care
   6. Encourage exercise to prevent constipation; administer laxatives as needed
   7. Give help in a matter-of-fact manner
   8. Assess the risk of suicide
   9. Observe for medication compliance and side effects

F. Nursing interventions: Behavioral needs
   1. Mobilize the client to productive activity by assigning therapeutic tasks
   2. Provide opportunities for increased involvement in activities through a structured, daily program
   3. Select activities that ensure success and accomplishment
   4. Provide opportunities for exercise

G. Nursing interventions: Cognitive needs
   1. Increase self-esteem and sense of control over behavior
   2. Modify negative expectations and explore the extent of negative thinking
   3. Substitute positive thoughts for negative

4. Establish realistic goals

H. Nursing interventions: Emotional needs
   1. Slowly and cautiously make the client aware of unconscious feelings
   2. Plan activities that allow for physical sublimation of aggressive feelings
   3. Talk about the universality of feelings
   4. Encourage constructive expression when the client discusses anger
   5. Provide hope
   6. Assess yourself: depression can be contagious

I. Nursing interventions: Spiritual needs
   1. Assess the client's loss of belief
   2. Help the client explore spiritual beliefs or a meaningful philosophy of life
   3. Arrange for a spiritual advisor to visit, if appropriate

# VIII. Manic reactions

A. Assessment: Characteristics
   1. Condition that usually develops more rapidly than depressive reactions
   2. Failure to view behavior as inappropriate
   3. Maladaptive defense against depression

B. Assessment: Physical manifestations
   1. Deteriorated physical appearance
   2. Increased energy; feeling of being "charged up"
   3. Increased sexual interest and activity
   4. Decreased sleep disturbance

C. Assessment: Emotional manifestations
   1. Mood lability; euphoria
   2. Feelings of grandiosity
   3. Inflated sense of self-worth

D. Assessment: Cognitive manifestations
   1. Difficulty concentrating
   2. Flight of ideas
   3. Delusions of grandeur
   4. Impaired judgment

E. Assessment: Behavioral manifestations
   1. Pressured speech
   2. Hyperactivity
   3. Impulsiveness, lack of inhibition, recklessness
   4. Increased social contacts
   5. Hypersexuality
   6. Verbosity; often rhyming and punning
   7. Bizarre and eccentric appearance

F. Nursing care goals
1. Prevent the client from self-harm
2. Decrease disorientation, delusions, bizarre behavior and dress, sexual acting-out, hyperactivity, restlessness, agitation
3. Promote rest, sleep, and a nutritious diet
4. Assist with activities of daily living
5. Provide emotional support
6. Promote medication compliance

G. Nursing interventions: Physical needs
1. Decrease environmental stimuli by acting as a consistent caregiver who supplies external controls
2. Offer finger foods
3. Encourage short rest periods
4. Enforce minimal standards of personal hygiene
5. Monitor medications

H. Nursing interventions: Behavioral needs
1. Suggest sedentary activities, and offer motor activities in moderation
2. Define and explain acceptable behaviors, then set limits
3. Negotiate limits on demanding, manipulative behaviors
4. Avoid frustrating the client unnecessarily

I. Nursing interventions: Cognitive needs
1. Safeguard the client from physical risks
2. Discourage the client from expensive purchases
3. Help the client identify behaviors that lead to a manic episode
4. Explore effects of behavior on others
5. Intervene when the client has DELUSIONS
6. Increase the client's self-esteem

J. Nursing interventions: Emotional needs
1. Help the client become aware of underlying anger
2. Verbally acknowledge resistance to therapy
3. Teach the client to make decisions and accept responsibility

K. Nursing interventions: Spiritual needs
1. Help the client explore a meaningful philosophy of life
2. Arrange for a spiritual advisor to visit, if appropriate

# IX. Evaluation

A. Use observation and the client's reports as a basis for evaluation

B. Note goal accomplishment

C. Note client growth in insight and development of alternate coping skills

D. Keep in mind the depressed client's reluctance to acknowledge progress

E. Complete a nursing self-assessment

## Points to remember

Alterations in mood are common responses to life changes.

Mood disorders are maladaptive responses to loss characterized by extreme disturbances in affect.

No single etiology of mood disorders has been universally accepted or empirically validated.

All clients with mood disorders should be assessed for suicide risk.

Nursing care goals and interventions vary, depending on the client and the disorder, and should be carefully individualized following assessment.

## Glossary

The following terms are defined in Appendix A, page 142.

affect

delusions

depression

mania

## Study questions

To evaluate your understanding of this chapter, answer the following questions in the space provided; then compare your responses with the correct answers in Appendix B, pages 151 and 152.

1. What are the five biologic etiologies for mood disorders? _____

   _____

2. Who developed the learned helplessness concept as an etiology for mood disorders? _____

   _____

3. What are the six special treatment measures for mood disorders? _____

   _____

   _____

4. Which cognitive changes will the nurse observe when a client is experiencing
   moderate depression?_____

   _____

5. When a client is experiencing depression, which nursing intervention is most
   important in meeting the client's physical needs?_____

   _____

6. What are the primary nursing care goals when caring for a manic client?

   _____

   _____

## CHAPTER 9

# Suicide

## Learning objectives

Check off the following items once you've mastered them:

☐ Describe eight common myths of suicide.

☐ Identify groups at high risk for suicidal behavior.

☐ Describe the physical, emotional, cognitive, and behavioral characteristics of a suicidal individual.

☐ Complete a nursing assessment of a suicidal client.

☐ Formulate a nursing care plan for a hospitalized suicidal client.

# I. Introduction

A. The ultimate form of self-destructive behavior, suicide is condemned in most societies and illegal in some states

B. Depending on its severity, suicidal behavior can take the form of a threat, a gesture, or an attempt

C. Suicidal intent is commonly signaled by mood swings, decline in job performance, and withdrawal from family and friends

D. Suicide is not necessarily the act of someone who is mentally ill

# II. Epidemiology

A. Statistics reflect incomplete reporting

B. More women than men attempt suicide

C. More men than women are successful

D. Suicide accounts for 1% of all deaths each year

E. It is the 10th leading cause of death for all ages and the 4th leading cause of death between ages 10 and 24

F. The suicide rate is increasing among elderly persons and teenagers

G. Incidence is higher in urban areas

H. Suicide tends to be seasonal, with the highest number occurring in April and May and the lowest in December

I. Suicide occurs most frequently on Fridays, Sundays, and Mondays

J. It is 500 times more prevalent among people with serious depressive reactions

# III. Myths about suicide

A. People who talk about suicide don't do it

B. Suicide happens without warning

C. Suicidal people wish to die

D. Once someone becomes suicidal, the person is always suicidal

E. Once a person's depression has lifted, the danger of suicide is over

F. Suicide is inherited and runs in families

G. Suicidal people are mentally ill

H. If someone is despondent, mentioning suicide will give the person suicidal ideas

## IV. Theories of suicidal behavior

A. Psychological
   1. Hostile feelings turned inward
   2. Loss of self-esteem resulting from self-condemnation and guilt
   3. Ego withdrawal resulting from stress
   4. Attempt to gain immortality, maintain ego, or solve an identification conflict

B. Biological
   1. Extreme confusion or personality disorganization related to organic brain disorders, PSYCHOSIS, or drug ingestion
   2. Behavior whose complications are commonly unrecognized by the person involved

C. Socioeconomic
   1. Painful or life-threatening illness
   2. Inadequate integration into society

D. Communication
   1. Form of communication or aggressive retaliation
   2. Way of relieving guilt

E. Sociopsychological
   1. Result of unsatisfactory relationships or breakup of satisfactory relationships
   2. Outcome of unsatisfactory social interaction
   3. Effort to solve problems of living

## V. Nursing assessment: High-risk groups

A. Alcoholics

B. Police officers

C. Physicians

D. Those with previous attempts

E. Adolescents

F. Terminally ill persons

G. Accident repeaters

H. Elderly persons

I. People who reject treatment

J. Medically ignored persons

K. Minority groups

L. Psychotics

## VI. Nursing assessment: Client behaviors and dynamics

A. Physical manifestations
   1. Depression in about 75% of cases
   2. Vague, nonspecific somatic complaints

B. Emotional manifestations
   1. Worthlessness
   2. Helplessness
   3. Hopelessness
   4. Ambivalence
   5. Anxiety
   6. Fear
   7. Excessive guilt
   8. Self-blame
   9. Frustration
   10. Anger
   11. Emotional calmness

C. Cognitive manifestations
   1. Preoccupation with self-harm
   2. Desire to escape untenable life situation
   3. DICHOTOMOUS THINKING
   4. SEMANTIC FALLACIES (for example, "Tom ignored me; that must mean I'm no good")

D. Behavioral manifestations
   1. Sudden behavioral changes
   2. Decision to put affairs in order
   3. Disclosure of coded or direct messages (for example, "I won't be seeing you again")

## VII. Nursing assessment: Stressors and risk factors

A. Age
   1. 45 or older
   2. Adolescents

B. Sex: male

C. Marital status
   1. Divorced
   2. Widowed
   3. Separated

D. Socialization: isolated

E. Occupation
   1. Professionals
   2. Students

F. Unemployment

G. Chronic or terminal illness

H. Mental illness
   1. Depression
   2. Delusions
   3. Hallucinations

I. Drug and alcohol use
   1. Intoxication
   2. Addiction

J. Previous suicide attempts

K. Well-developed plan with available means

## VIII. Nursing assessment: Additional factors

A. Level of intent

B. Plan
   1. Lethality of planned method
   2. Availability of means
   3. Concreteness and completeness of plan
   4. Precise preparations for death

C. Verbal clues

D. Psychological state

E. Expression of feelings

F. Community support systems

G. Medical status

## IX. Diagnoses

A. *DSM-III-R* medical diagnoses
   1. Bipolar disorder, depressed
   2. Bipolar disorder, mixed
   3. Borderline personality disorder
   4. Hallucinogen mood disorder
   5. Major depression, single or recurrent episode
   6. Multi-infarct dementia with depression
   7. Organic mood syndrome
   8. Phencyclidine (PCP) or similarly acting arylcyclohexylamine (hallucinogen-induced) mood disorder
   9. Primary DEGENERATIVE DEMENTIA of the Alzheimer type with depression
   10. SCHIZOAFFECTIVE DISORDER

B. Primary NANDA diagnostic categories
   1. Ineffective individual coping
   2. Fear
   3. Dysfunctional grieving
   4. Self-esteem disturbance
   5. Altered family processes
   6. Social isolation
   7. Altered role performance
   8. Noncompliance
   9. Potential for self-directed violence

## X. Treatment modalities

A. Outpatient crisis intervention

B. Inpatient hospitalization

C. Pharmacology
   1. Antidepressant agents
   2. Antianxiety agents
   3. Antimanic agents

D. Electroconvulsive therapy

## XI. Nursing care goals and interventions for the hospitalized client

A. Provide a safe environment, and protect the client from self-harm
   1. Determine the appropriate level of suicide precautions, and explain them to the client
   2. Assess the client's suicide potential daily
   3. Evaluate the level of precautions daily
   4. Obtain assessment data in a matter-of-fact manner
   5. Ask the client directly about the suicide plan
   6. Remove dangerous objects
   7. Place the client in a room near the nurses' station, in view of staff
   8. Make sure the windows are locked
   9. Stay with the client when sharp objects must be used

B. Maintain close supervision
   1. Know the whereabouts of the client at all times
   2. Stay with the client during bathing, shaving, and similar activities
   3. Check the client at frequent, irregular intervals at night
   4. Be especially alert when the staff is reduced (change of shift, holidays, weekends)
   5. Observe and note behavior patterns
   6. Be aware of manipulative or attention-seeking behavior

C. Be alert to the possibility that the client is either saving or not taking medications
   1. Observe and report sudden changes in mood; a sudden calmness or lifting of depression may indicate that the client has decided on suicide and formulated a plan
   2. Avoid promising not to tell
   3. Watch for decreased communication, conversations about death, disorientation, dependency, or concealing of articles

D. Place limits on RUMINATION about suicide; discuss the client's emotions but not the previous attempts

E. Prevent the client from harming others

F. Promote adequate nutrition, hydration, and elimination

G. Promote a balance of rest, sleep, and activity

H. Reduce feelings of depression; encourage feelings of self-worth
   1. Convey caring
   2. Encourage the client to express feelings
   3. Do not joke about death
   4. Do not belittle previous attempts
   5. Provide opportunities for successful accomplishment of tasks or goals to enhance the client's self-worth
   6. Help the client identify positive aspects of the self
   7. Involve the client, if possible, in planning treatment

I. Reduce withdrawal from people
   1. Seek out the client for conversation
   2. Encourage the client to spend time away from the hospital room
   3. Promote group interaction as appropriate

J. Help the client develop insight and a willingness to express feelings
   1. Encourage and support expressions of feelings
   2. Examine the client's relationships with others

K. Increase the client's ability to deal with future suicidal feelings
   1. Review hypothetical situations
   2. Plan how to recognize and deal with feelings and situations that have caused stress

L. Complete a nursing self-assessment

## XII. Nursing care goals and interventions for families following suicide

A. Lessen long-term effects and promote grieving

B. Recognize that support from friends is commonly lacking

C. Help the family explore their guilt

D. Be alert to an "anniversary suicide" by a survivor

E. Help the family deal with hostility and destructiveness

## XIII. Evaluation

A. Psychological autopsy (review of the client's life to determine whether anything could have been done to prevent suicide)

B. Nursing self-assessment

## Points to remember

Suicide is more prevalent among those with severe depressive reactions; suicide is not necessarily the act of someone who mentally ill.

Common characteristics of suicidal persons are ambivalence, guilt, helplessness, hopelessness, loneliness, and a lack of future orientation.

The major nursing care goal for a suicidal client is to provide a safe environment while protecting the client from self-harm.

The nurse must be prepared to ask direct questions about the client's suicidal thoughts and plans.

## Glossary

The following terms are defined in Appendix A, page 142.

degenerative dementia                   rumination

dichotomous thinking                    semantic fallacies

psychosis                               schizoaffective disorder

## Study questions

To evaluate your understanding of this chapter, answer the following questions in the space provided; then compare your responses with the correct answers in Appendix B, page 152.

1. Which groups are at high risk for suicide? _____

_____

2. What are the three categories of pharmacologic agents used to treat suicidal clients? _____

_____

3. Which methods would a nurse use to create a safe environment and protect the client from harm? _____

_____

4. Which nursing goals and interventions are important when caring for the families of a suicide victim? _____

_____

## CHAPTER 10

# Alteration in Thought and Perception: Schizophrenia

## Learning objectives

Check off the following items once you've mastered them:

☐ Define psychotic behavior.

☐ Describe four theories that explain the etiology of schizophrenia.

☐ Describe four manifestations of various types of schizophrenia.

☐ Identify nursing diagnoses appropriate to the schizophrenic client.

☐ Develop a nursing care plan for the schizophrenic client.

# I. Introduction

A. PSYCHOTIC BEHAVIOR includes various symptoms resulting from disturbed thought processes, distorted PERCEPTIONS, brain damage, or chemical toxicity

B. Schizophrenia is a group of disorders manifested by changes in the cognitive, perceptual, affective, motor, and social domains

C. The psychotic person perceives reality differently from most people and has difficulty evaluating it

D. Schizophrenia can be characterized by remissions and exacerbations

E. Health experts do not universally agree on the diagnosis, etiology, or treatment of schizophrenia

F. Schizophrenic clients experience a split between thought and affect and a split with reality

# II. Etiology

A. General comments
   1. Current explanations, which remain inconclusive, are based on interactions among factors
   2. Considerable laboratory data support biochemical causes

B. Genetic theories
   1. Biological relatives of persons with schizophrenia are at greater risk
   2. Vulnerability increases with closeness of biological relationship
   3. Monogenic theory assumes transmission of a single gene that produces susceptibility to schizophrenia; under stress, the carrier is likely to become schizophrenic
   4. Polygenic theory assumes causation by inheritance of more than one gene
   5. Social or environmental stress may contribute to the disorder's onset by interacting with the person's inherited biological makeup

C. Biochemical theories
   1. Schizophrenia is caused by physiologic dysfunction
   2. No dominant causative factor has been established
   3. Research points to bioamine transmission as a likely factor
   4. Toxic blood substances have been linked to abnormal brain chemistry and aberrant behaviors
   5. Two current hypotheses under investigation are the TRANSMETHYLATION hypothesis and the dopamine hypothesis
      a. The *transmethylation hypothesis* suggests a link between schizophrenia and abnormal transmethylation of catecholamines; this abnormality leads to the production of dimethoxyphenylthelyla- mine (DMPEA), which is similar to mescaline

b. The *dopamine hypothesis* suggests a link between schizophrenia and excess dopamine; this excess results in overactivity of neurons

D. Developmental theories
1. The disorder starts early in life when the relationship between the child and the primary caregiver is impaired or inadequate
2. Deficient nurturing results in difficulty learning to interact with others and an inability to trust oneself or others
3. The theory focuses on the child's need to receive and give love
4. The child is traumatized by a lack or an unpredictability of maternal love
5. Symbiotic relationships prevent normal maturation
6. Schizophrenogenic mothers have been described as overinvolved, yet anxious, ungiving, and unpredictable
7. Schizophrenogenic fathers have been described as weak, ineffectual role models
8. In schizophrenogenic families, relationships are intricate and confusing

E. Psychodynamic theories
1. Schizophrenia may be preceded by the formation of a fragile ego, which cannot withstand the demands of external reality
2. Conflicts arise when a disparity exists between psychological needs and sociocultural expectations
3. The relationship with the mother is marked by ambivalence
4. Difficulty separating from the mother may be a factor in the disorder's onset

## III. Sequential steps of the schizophrenic process

A. Inability to trust

B. Dissociation

C. Displacement

D. Fantasy

E. Projection

## IV. Assessment: Primary manifestations

A. Associative looseness
1. Inability to organize thoughts logically
2. Inability to pursue a single concept to a logical conclusion
3. Unrelated thoughts
4. Irrelevant ideas
5. Magical thinking

B. AUTISTIC THINKING
1. Form of subjective thinking
2. Reliance on a personal and illogical interpretation of reality
3. Minimal distinction between the self and the environment
4. Thinking not validated by objective reality
5. Fantasy and daydreaming as substitutes for reality
6. Personal meanings applied to persons and events

C. Ambivalence
1. Conflicting feelings toward self, significant others, situations, events, and relationships
2. Negativism; repetitious, ceaseless, nonmeaningful activity; overcompliance; apathy; or immobilization

D. Alterations of affect
1. Protective actions
2. Inappropriate affect: outward display is not in harmony with reality
3. Blunted affect: extreme decrease in the intensity of response
4. Apathy: indifference to the environment characterized by a lack of commitment and involvement

## V. Assessment: Cognitive manifestations

A. Concrete thinking

B. Blocked speech

C. Poverty of speech and ideas

D. Symbolic associations

E. TANGENTIALITY

F. Stereotyped speech

G. DELUSIONS
1. May include grandeur, persecution, reference, influence, and somatic types
2. Develop through stages of anxiety, denial, projection, and rationalization
3. Reflect an underlying need to deny unacceptable feelings about the self

## VI. Assessment: Linguistic manifestations

A. ECHOLALIA

B. CLANG ASSOCIATION

C. NEOLOGISM

D. WORD SALAD

E. MUTISM

## VII. Assessment: Perceptual manifestations (hallucinations)

A. Are false sensory perceptions with no basis in reality, generated by internal rather than external stimuli

B. Include auditory, gustatory, olfactory, tactile, visual, and somatic hallucinations

C. Develop in three phases
   1. The client focuses on comforting thoughts to relieve anxiety and stress
   2. The client projects these thoughts to external objects
   3. The client experiences increasing preoccupation and helplessness; the hallucination is controlling but comforting, although content may become menacing

D. May become chronic if no intervention occurs

## VIII. Assessment: Affective manifestations

A. Overresponse

B. Blunted AFFECT

C. Lack of affect

D. Lability

## IX. Assessment: Alterations in body image

A. Depersonalization
   1. Lack of ego boundaries
   2. Feelings of unreality and instability about the self
   3. Sense of living in a dream
   4. Inability to discriminate between the inner and outer parts of one's body
   5. Loss of self-control
   6. Sense of merging with the environment

B. Identity confusion
   1. Loss of orientation in space
   2. Inability to recognize sexual identity

C. Hypochondriasis
   1. Intense self-focus
   2. Preoccupation with bodily sensations and functions
   3. Physical symptoms with no basis in reality

## X. Assessment: Behavioral manifestations

A. Withdrawal

B. Regression

C. Overactivity or underactivity

D. Impulsivity

E. Mannerisms

F. Automatism

G. Stereotypy (rigid categorization or structure)

## XI. Assessment: Social manifestations

A. Anxiety associated with relatedness (ability to establish intimate relationships) plus autistic thinking

B. Loneliness
  1. Estrangement
  2. Emptiness, barrenness, and despair

C. Social isolation
  1. Intense shyness to complete reclusiveness
  2. Dependent on the degree of anxiety generated by interaction

D. Superficial relationships
  1. Mistrust of others
  2. Perception of others as inauthentic, unreliable, and dangerous

E. Dependence
  1. Excessive reliance on others
  2. Attempts to manipulate others by repeated demands

## XII. Problem and need identification

A. Priority problems commonly relate to basic physical and safety needs in an acute psychotic episode

B. Problems are interrelated; the etiology of one problem may, in itself, be a separate problem

C. Not all symptoms are separate problems

D. Problems should be grouped in related concepts

## XIII. Diagnoses

A. *DSM-III-R* medical diagnostic types
  1. Disorganized
  2. Catatonic
  3. Paranoid
  4. Undifferentiated
  5. Residual

B. Primary NANDA diagnostic categories
  1. Ineffective individual coping

      2. Self-esteem disturbance
      3. Social isolation
      4. Altered thought process
  C. Secondary NANDA diagnostic categories
      1. Anxiety
      2. Sensory-perceptual alteration
      3. Impaired social interaction
      4. Self-care deficit
      5. Impaired verbal communication
      6. Potential for self-injury
      7. Potential for injury to others

# XIV. Treatment modalities

  A. Psychopharmacology
      1. Neuroleptics (antipsychotics)
      2. Antiparkinsonian medications (for side effects of neuroleptics)

  B. RELATIONSHIP THERAPY

  C. Group therapy

  D. Individual psychotherapy

  E. MILIEU THERAPY

  F. Family therapy

# XV. Implementing nursing care

  A. Unless educationally prepared to conduct group or family therapy, the nurse generalist uses relationship therapy

  B. Nurse must convey a sincere wish to understand and communicate

  C. Principles of therapeutic interaction include:
      1. Acceptance of client
      2. Acknowledgment
      3. Authenticity
      4. Self-awareness

  D. Trust is essential to effective nursing care

# XVI. Nursing care goals and interventions

  A. Provide a safe environment
      1. Briefly explain procedures, routines, and tests
      2. Protect the client from self-destructive tendencies

  B. Monitor physical needs; maintain adequate nutrition, hydration, and elimination

C. Decrease withdrawn behavior
1. Spend time with the client
2. Do not make unrealistic promises
3. Teach the client that feelings are valid
4. Limit the client's environment
5. Maintain staff consistency
6. Begin with one-on-one interactions, then progress to small groups
7. Establish a daily routine

D. Increase the client's self-esteem
1. Provide attention in a sincere manner
2. Offer praise
3. Avoid trying to convince the client of worth verbally
4. Assist with activities of daily living

E. Orient the client to reality

F. Help the client establish ego boundaries
1. Validate the client's real perceptions
2. Correct misconceptions in a matter-of-fact manner
3. Do not argue
4. Stay with the frightened client
5. Discuss simple, concrete topics
6. Provide activities that maintain contact with reality

G. Maintain a safe, therapeutic environment for other clients
1. Remove the client from the group when necessary
2. Help the group accept the client's behavior
3. Make sure that at least one staff member attends to other clients
4. Explain to other clients that the client's behavior is a result of illness and not of anything they did

H. Help the client work through regressive behavior
1. Assess the present level of functioning, and communicate with the client at that level
2. Encourage more adult behavior
3. Help identify unmet needs or feelings
4. Encourage the expression of feelings
5. Set realistic goals and expectations daily
6. Make the client aware of expectations
7. Initially, make choices for the client
8. Gradually, offer the client opportunities to make decisions and accept responsibility

I. Reduce bizarre behavior, anxiety, agitation, or aggression
1. Set limits on behavior
2. Reduce excessive stimuli
3. Give medication as needed

## XVII. Intervening in delusions

A. Provide sensitivity

B. Avoid supporting or reinforcing the delusion

C. Do not directly attack the delusion; this will increase anxiety

D. Express doubt tactfully

E. Recognize delusion as the client's perception of the environment

F. Focus on reality

G. Avoid judging

H. Empathize with the client's feelings and help the person deal with underlying needs or feelings in a healthy way

I. Maintain homeostasis

## XVIII. Intervening in hallucinations

A. Assess the underlying unmet need

B. Establish trust

C. Recognize and acknowledge the affective component

D. Be alert for clues that the client is hallucinating

E. Cast doubt tactfully

F. Discuss reality-based issues

G. Protect the client from self-harm or harm to others or objects

H. Reduce stimuli

I. Communicate in direct, concrete, specific terms

J. Provide simple activities

K. Evaluate the client's ability to tolerate touch

L. Provide a structured environment

M. Assess signs of increasing fear, anxiety, or agitation

N. Intervene appropriately (for example, with one-on-one contact, seclusion, medication)

O. Do not corner the client

P. Help the client express feelings

Q. Help the client deal with guilt, remorse, or embarrassment when he remembers psychotic behavior

R. Help the client deal with possible recurrence of hallucinations

## XIX. Evaluation

    A. Document progress for the client

    B. Be realistic; expect change to be slow

    C. Modify the care plan as needed

    D. Complete a self-evaluation

## Points to remember

Statistics on the incidence and prevalence of schizophrenia are unreliable because of disagreements about diagnosis.

Etiologic explanations of schizophrenia remain inconclusive.

Primary symptoms of altered patterns of thought and perception include ambivalence, autism, altered affect, and loose associations.

The use of major tranquilizers has enabled many schizophrenics to participate in other therapies and to function outside the hospital.

Relationship therapy is the most suitable therapy for generalist nurses working with schizophrenic clients.

## Glossary

The following terms are defined in Appendix A, page 142.

| | |
|---|---|
| affect | neologism |
| autistic thinking | perceptions |
| clang association | psychotic behavior |
| delusions | relationship therapy |
| echolalia | tangentiality |
| milieu therapy | transmethylation |
| mutism | word salad |

## Study questions

To evaluate your understanding of this chapter, answer the following questions in the space provided; then compare your responses with the correct answers in Appendix B, pages 152 and 153.

1. What is psychotic behavior? _____

_____

2. What are the sequential steps of the schizophrenic process? _____

_____

3. Which primary manifestations are identified during assessment of a client with schizophrenia? _____

_____

4. How do perceptual manifestations (hallucinations) develop? _____

_____

5. What are four behavioral manifestations that the nurse might see when assessing the client with schizophrenia? _____

_____

6. What is the priority problem in an acute psychotic episode? _____

_____

7. What are the principles of therapeutic interaction? _____

_____

8. How would a nurse help a client establish ego boundaries? _____

_____

## CHAPTER 11

# Disruptions in Social Relatedness: Personality Disorders

## Learning objectives

Check off the following items once you've mastered them:

☐ Identify at least six characteristics of a healthy interpersonal relationship.

☐ Discuss the four predisposing factors that contribute to disruptions in relatedness.

☐ Describe six behaviors associated with each of four personality disorders.

☐ Formulate individualized nursing diagnoses for clients with personality disorders.

☐ Develop a nursing care plan for clients with personality disorders.

# I. Characteristics of healthy interpersonal relationships

A. Intimacy while maintaining separate identities

B. Sensitivity to needs of another

C. Mutual validation of personal worth

D. Open communication of feelings

E. Acceptance of another as a valued, separate person

F. Deep EMPATHY

G. Willingness to risk self-revelation

H. Ability and willingness to subordinate one's needs to those of another or to the demands of a relationship

I. Interdependency

J. EGO-SYNTONIC BEHAVIOR

# II. Development of relatedness throughout the life cycle

A. Infancy
1. Infant depends on others
2. Trust develops as a result of a consistent, reliable relationship with a significant other

B. Childhood
1. The child strives to establish the self as a separate individual
2. Parental love and consistent limit-setting communicate caring
3. The child develops a capacity for interdependence
4. Parental guidelines for behavior are internalized
5. A value system emerges
6. Peer relationships and approval of adults outside the family group become important

C. Preadolescence and adolescence
1. The child experiences intimate, dependent, same-sex relationships
2. Dependent heterosexual relationships appear
3. Independence from parents increases
4. The child balances parental demands and peer group pressure

D. Young adulthood
1. Interdependent relationships form
2. The young adult makes independent decisions
3. Occupational plans are implemented
4. Dependent and independent behaviors are balanced
5. Sensitivity to and acceptance of feelings and needs of the self and others increase
6. Interpersonal relationships are characterized by mutuality

E. Middle adulthood
   1. Independence is fostered in others, such as children
   2. Self-reliance increases
   3. Interdependent relationship with children is established

F. Late adulthood
   1. The adult experiences and deals with losses
   2. New relationships develop
   3. Cultural contributions continue or increase
   4. As much independence as possible is retained, but increased dependence is accepted

## III. Predisposing factors

A. Developmental factors
   1. Any unaccomplished developmental task
   2. Disrupted relationship with the mothering person

B. Family communication factors
   1. Disruptive relationships manifested in symptomatic behavior of one member
   2. Deviant behavior when the family is highly stressed
   3. Closed family system that discourages relationships with others

C. Sociocultural factors
   1. Mores against casual acquaintances
   2. Mobility that contributes to transient friendships
   3. Social isolation, especially among elderly, handicapped, and chronically ill persons
   4. Romanticization of heterosexual relationships

## IV. Dependency and helplessness

A. Characteristics
   1. Fear and anxiety
   2. Hypersensitivity to potential rejection
   3. Passive relinquishing of control
   4. Indirect RESISTANCE to occupational and social performance
   5. Clinging, demanding behavior

B. *DSM-III-R* medical diagnoses: Paranoid personality disorder
   1. Avoidant personality disorder
   2. Dependent personality disorder
   3. Passive-aggressive personality disorders

C. Nursing interventions
   1. Anticipate the client's needs before they demand attention
   2. Set realistic limits
   3. Help the client manage anxiety

4. Teach the client to express ideas and feelings assertively
5. Support the client in accepting increased decision making
6. Clarify roles

## V. Suspiciousness

A. Characteristics
   1. Distrust
   2. Rigidity
   3. Expectations of trickery or harm
   4. Secretiveness
   5. Guardedness
   6. Jealousy
   7. Overconcern with hidden motives
   8. Hypersensitivity and hyperalertness
   9. Distortions of reality
   10. PROJECTION

B. *DSM-III-R* medical diagnosis: Paranoid personality disorder

C. Nursing interventions
   1. Overcome the client's lack of insight and rigidity of thoughts
   2. Reestablish communication and FEEDBACK with the client
   3. Reduce social isolation
   4. Keep messages clear and consistent
   5. Avoid pretense and deception
   6. Provide CONSENSUAL VALIDATION
   7. Foster trust
   8. Minimize anxiety
   9. Provide environmental support
   10. Respect privacy

## VI. Withdrawal

A. Characteristics
   1. Incapable of forming warm, tender relationships
   2. Indifferent to praise, criticisms, and feelings of others
   3. Reclusive
   4. Vague about goals
   5. Indecisive
   6. Detached

B. *DSM-III-R* medical diagnoses
   1. Schizoid personality disorder
   2. Schizotypal personality disorder

C. Nursing interventions
   1. Attend to basic daily needs
   2. Establish therapeutic interpersonal communication

3. Enhance social interactions with others
4. Establish realistic goals
5. Use consistent, repeated approaches

# VII. Impulsivity and manipulation

A. Characteristics
1. Inability to form significant loyalties or close, lasting relationships
2. Selfishness
3. Inability to delay gratification
4. Superficial charm and above-average intelligence
5. Unreliability
6. Insincerity
7. Lack of remorse, shame, guilt, or anxiety except under external stress
8. Inadequate motivation
9. Poor judgment
10. Failure to learn by experience
11. Egocentricity
12. Specific loss of insight
13. Failure to follow a life plan
14. Inability to tolerate frustration
15. Manipulativeness

B. *DSM-III-R* medical diagnoses
1. Antisocial personality disorder
2. Borderline personality disorder

C. Nursing interventions
1. Overcome lack of motivation to change
2. Provide model of mature behavior
3. Assist in developing positive relationships
4. Convey concern and interest
5. Assist with problem solving
6. Encourage fewer acting-out behaviors
7. Facilitate verbal communication
8. Support personal developmental growth
9. Anticipate and deal with depression
10. Set limits on manipulative behavior
11. Control personal resentment

# VIII. Treatment modalities

A. Antianxiety medications

B. Behavior modification

C. Individual psychotherapy

## Points to remember

Altered patterns of social relatedness are functional disturbances of personality.

Personality disorders are lifelong behavior patterns that are acceptable to the individual but that create conflict with others.

A combination of predisposing developmental, family communication, and sociocultural factors contributes to the development of personality disorders.

Treatment is difficult because clients with personality disorders lack motivation to change.

Nursing interventions for clients with personality disorders require self-awareness and action rather than reaction.

## Glossary

The following terms are defined in Appendix A, page 142.

| | |
|---|---|
| consensual validation | feedback |
| ego-syntonic behavior | projection |
| empathy | resistance |

## Study questions

To evaluate your understanding of this chapter, answer the following questions in the space provided; then compare your responses with the correct answers in Appendix B, page 153.

1. What are the characteristics of healthy interpersonal relationships? _____

_____

_____

2. Which steps does a young adult take in developing relatedness? _____

_____

_____

3. What can a nurse do if a client experiences dependency and helplessness?

_____

_____

4. What is the key characteristic of a client experiencing suspiciousness?

_____

_____

5. What nursing diagnosis would likely apply to a client who is incapable of forming warm, tender relationships? _____

_____

6. Which treatment modalities can a nurse use for a client with a personality disorder? _____

_____

## CHAPTER 12

# Substance Abuse

## Learning objectives

Check off the following items once you've mastered them:

☐ Identify five patterns of substance use and behavioral patterns of substance abusers.

☐ Discuss six predisposing factors of substance abuse.

☐ Compare and contrast the eight major categories of abused substances.

☐ Formulate individualized nursing diagnoses appropriate for substance abuse disorders.

☐ Develop a nursing care plan for clients in the acute and rehabilitative phases of substance abuse.

# I. Introduction
   A. Individuals who abuse drugs develop altered patterns of social adjustment

   B. Drugs of any type can be misused

   C. Alcohol is a drug

# II. Terminology
   A. Abuse
     1. Use that interferes with the individual's biological, psychological, or sociocultural functioning
     2. A pervasive disorder
     3. Use that differs from approved medical or social patterns

   B. TOLERANCE

   C. Physical dependence

   D. Withdrawal symptoms
     1. Physical disturbances that occur when use of a drug ceases
     2. Rebound effects occurring in the same physiologic system

   E. PSYCHOLOGICAL DEPENDENCE

   F. Addiction
     1. Preoccupation with compulsive use
     2. Preoccupation with securing supply
     3. Tendency to renewed addiction after withdrawal
     4. Behavior distinct from physical dependence

# III. Patterns of substance use
   A. Experimental

   B. Recreational

   C. Circumstantial
     1. Used to cope with life's problems
     2. Carries potential for abuse

   D. Intensified
     1. Heavy, frequent use
     2. Abuse

   E. Compulsive
     1. High frequency
     2. High intensity
     3. Abuse
     4. Dependence

## IV. Behavioral patterns of substance abusers

A. Dysfunctional anger

B. Manipulation
1. Attempts to meet needs by influencing others
2. Typically follows negative pattern of interaction
3. Deceives
4. Makes others feel used, powerless, and angry

C. Impulsiveness
1. Directs behaviors toward immediate gratification
2. Acts abruptly
3. May be active or passive
4. Uses impulses to avoid conscious feelings of guilt and anger

D. Avoidance
1. Facilitates an escape from anxiety associated with relatedness
2. Is characterized by running away or emotional distancing
3. Used to exert control

E. Grandiosity
1. Exalted or superior state
2. Denial and rationalization of the consequences of behavior
3. Commonly manifested by an unshakable belief in personal cleverness

## V. Predisposing factors

A. Biological factors
1. Familial tendency
2. Allergic response (not documented)
3. Vitamin deficiencies

B. Psychological factors (personality traits)
1. Dependent personality
2. Low self-esteem
3. Anger and frustration
4. Feelings of omnipotence
5. Depression
6. Defense mechanisms

C. Familial characteristics
1. History of multigenerational addictive behavior
2. Primitive and direct expression of conflict
3. Absence of schizophrenic behavior in parents
4. High level of maternal symbiosis
5. Presence of death themes and untimely deaths
6. Immigrant parents

D. Sociocultural factors
  1. Acceptance by relevant sociocultural group
  2. Failure to assimilate values opposing drug use
  3. Ambivalence of society
  4. Religious sanctions
  5. Cultural attitudes

E. Learning theory
  1. Reflex response aimed at reducing anxiety
  2. Peer and parental modeling
  3. Positive reinforcement provided by drugs

F. Disease model
  1. Chronic, progressive disorder
  2. Abuse caused by underlying physical or psychological disorder

## VI. Epidemiology

A. About 7% of adults in the United States are alcoholics

B. Nearly 95% of the adult population has tried alcohol at least once by age 25

C. Approximately 3.3 million alcohol abusers between ages 14 and 17 are problem drinkers

D. Alcohol is involved in more than one-third of all suicides

E. More than 15% of adults use depressants

F. About 0.5% of the U.S. population is addicted to narcotics

## VII. Commonly abused drugs

A. Alcohol

B. Stimulants
  1. Amphetamines
  2. Cocaine
  3. Caffeine

C. Opiates and related analgesics
  1. Heroin
  2. Morphine
  3. Codeine
  4. Hydromorphone
  5. Oxycodone
  6. Methadone
  7. Meperidine
  8. Diphenoxylate
  9. Pentazocine
  10. Combination of heroin and cocaine taken intravenously

D. Depressants
   1. Hypnotics
   2. Antianxiety drugs
   3. Barbiturates

E. Marijuana (cannabis)

F. Hallucinogens
   1. Lysergic acid diethylamide (LSD)
   2. Psilocybin
   3. Mescaline
   4. Phencyclidine (PCP)
   5. 2,5-dimethoxy-4-methylamphetamine (STP)

G. Inhalants
   1. Glue
   2. Cleaning solutions
   3. Nail polish remover
   4. Aerosols
   5. Petroleum products
   6. Paint thinners

H. Designer drugs
   1. Crack
   2. Ice
   3. China white

## VIII. Diagnoses

A. *DSM-III-R* medical diagnoses
   1. Alcohol dependence
   2. Alcohol abuse
   3. Amphetamine or similarly acting sympathomimetic dependence
   4. Amphetamine or similarly acting sympathomimetic abuse
   5. Cannabis dependence
   6. Cannabis abuse
   7. Cocaine dependence
   8. Cocaine abuse
   9. Hallucinogen dependence
   10. Hallucinogen abuse
   11. Inhalant dependence
   12. Inhalant abuse
   13. Nicotine dependence
   14. Opioid dependence
   15. Opioid abuse
   16. Phencyclidine (PCP) or similarly acting arylcyclohexylamine
       (hallucinogen-induced) dependence

17. Phencyclidine (PCP) or similarly acting arylcyclohexylamine (hallucinogen-induced) abuse
18. Sedative, hypnotic, or anxiolytic dependence
19. Sedative, hypnotic, or anxiolytic abuse
20. Multiple substance dependence
21. Psychoactive substance dependence (not otherwise specified)
22. Psychoactive substance abuse (not otherwise specified)

B. Primary NANDA diagnostic categories
1. Altered thought process
2. Sensory-perceptual alteration

C. Secondary NANDA diagnostic categories
1. Anxiety
2. Ineffective individual coping
3. Impaired social interaction
4. Potential for injury
5. Self-esteem disturbance
6. Sleep pattern disturbance
7. Potential for violence

D. Dual diagnoses
1. Meet criteria for at least one drug disorder and a mental illness
2. Thought to be more common than previously identified

# IX. Behaviors associated with alcoholism

A. Pre-alcoholic phase
1. Use of alcohol to relax
2. Increased tolerance

B. Early alcoholic phase
1. Sneaking of drinks
2. Denial of drinking
3. Blackouts

C. ADDICTION phase
1. Loss of control over drinking
2. Aggressive behavior
3. Blaming of others for altered relationships
4. Withdrawal symptoms

D. Chronic phase
1. Indulgence in unplanned sprees
2. Solitary drinking
3. Physical complications

E. Physiologic consequences
1. Blackouts
2. Pathologic intoxication

    3. Alcohol WITHDRAWAL SYNDROME
    4. Acute alcoholic hallucinosis
    5. Wernicke's syndrome
    6. Korsakoff's syndrome
    7. Alcoholic paranoia
    8. Liver damage
    9. Gout symptoms
   10. Alcoholic hepatitis
   11. Alcoholic cirrhosis
   12. Gastritis
   13. Gastric ulcers
   14. Pancreatitis
   15. Malnutrition
   16. Alcoholic cardiomyopathy
   17. Muscular myopathy
   18. Adrenocortical insufficiency
   19. Erection problems

F. Withdrawal behavior
    1. Begins shortly after drinking stops
    2. Lasts 5 to 7 days
    3. Signaled by anxiety, anorexia, insomnia, tremors, hyperalertness, mild disorientation
    4. May include alcoholic hallucinosis (auditory hallucinations lasting for several hours), alcohol withdrawal delirium, and generalized motor seizures

# X. Nursing care problems and interventions in acute stage of alcoholism

A. Withdrawal
    1. Monitor vital signs
    2. Observe for signs of seizures and impending alcohol withdrawal syndrome

B. Inadequate food and fluid intake
    1. Provide a high-protein diet
    2. Provide mineral and vitamin supplements
    3. Record fluid intake and output
    4. Test urine for specific gravity and stool for blood
    5. Encourage fluid intake

C. Risk of self-injury
    1. Provide supervision
    2. Remove potentially harmful items
    3. Reduce anxiety

D. Self-care deficit
   1. Assist with personal care
   2. Delay unnecessary procedures

E. Need for rest and relaxation
   1. Avoid sudden approaches
   2. Explain reasons for all tests and procedures
   3. Provide measures to induce sleep

F. Anxiety
   1. Provide antianxiety drugs, as ordered
   2. Explain reasons for all tests and procedures
   3. Orient the client to reality
   4. Encourage the client to vent fear and anger

## XI. Nursing care problems and interventions in rehabilitative stage of alcoholism

A. Denial of illness
   1. Help the client accept that drinking must stop
   2. Confront denial and manipulation

B. Failure to understand the disease
   1. Educate the client about alcoholism
   2. Teach the effects of abuse

C. Low self-esteem
   1. Engage the client in tasks that lead to success
   2. Explore areas of competence
   3. Express hope of arresting alcoholism

D. Loneliness
   1. Provide positive interpersonal experiences
   2. Help the client express needs directly
   3. Identify ways of alleviating loneliness

E. Low tolerance for frustration
   1. Explore methods of relieving tension and anxiety
   2. Assist in developing constructive coping skills

F. Possibility of relapse
   1. Complete discharge planning
   2. Inform the client of available support systems

## XII. Behaviors associated with drug abuse

A. Opiate abuse
   1. Mental and physical deterioration
   2. Inability to function productively
   3. Pursuit of illegal behavior

    4. Rapidly developed tolerance
    5. Decreased response to pain
    6. Respiratory depression
    7. Nausea
    8. Constriction of pupils
    9. Drowsiness
  10. Depressed pituitary functioning
  11. Slowed peristalsis
  12. Constipation
  13. Euphoria
  14. Apathy
  15. Detachment from reality
  16. Impaired judgment
  17. Uncomfortable (but not life-threatening) withdrawal symptoms
  18. Psychological addiction
  19. Physical dependence

B. Stimulant abuse
    1. Alertness
    2. Hyperactivity
    3. Irritability
    4. Insomnia
    5. Anorexia
    6. Weight loss
    7. Tachycardia
    8. Hypertension
    9. Psychological dependence
  10. Rapidly developed tolerance (within hours or days)
  11. Panic reactions
  12. Paranoid delusions
  13. Suspicion

C. Depressant abuse
    1. Lethargy
    2. Sleepiness
    3. Respiratory depression
    4. Circulatory depression
    5. Tolerance
    6. Withdrawal with abrupt cessation
    7. Temporary psychoses

D. Hallucinogen abuse
    1. Intensified sensory experiences
    2. Distortion of time and space
    3. Absence of addiction
    4. Impaired judgment
    5. Delusions

6. Hallucinations
7. Flashbacks
8. Antisocial behaviors

E. Marijuana abuse
   1. Altered state of awareness
   2. Relaxation
   3. Mild euphoria
   4. Slowed reflexes
   5. Reduced inhibitions
   6. Apathy
   7. Lack of motivation
   8. Fine tremors
   9. Decreased muscle strength
   10. Decreased coordination
   11. Absence of tolerance
   12. Absence of physical dependence

F. Inhalant abuse
   1. Euphoria
   2. Decreased inhibition
   3. Misperceptions or illusions
   4. Cloudiness of thought
   5. Drowsiness
   6. Rapidly developed tolerance
   7. Absence of withdrawal symptoms

# XIII. Physiologic consequences of drug abuse

A. Circulatory and respiratory complications
   1. Bacterial endocarditis
   2. Gangrene
   3. Thrombophlebitis
   4. Sclerosing of veins
   5. Intracranial hemorrhage
   6. Pulmonary embolism
   7. Respiratory infections
   8. Tuberculosis
   9. Pulmonary abcesses
   10. Acquired immunodeficiency syndrome (AIDS)

B. Hepatic complications

C. Gastrointestinal complications
   1. Severe and rapid weight loss
   2. Vitamin deficiencies
   3. Severe constipation
   4. Hemorrhoids

   D. Integumentary complications
      1.  Scarring
      2.  Abscesses
      3.  Cellulitis
      4.  Ulcerations

   E. Muscular complications
      1.  Fibrosing myopathy
      2.  Chronic muscle damage

   F. Other complications
      1.  Tetanus
      2.  Eye emboli
      3.  Traumatic injury

## XIV. Nursing care problems and interventions for acute drug reactions

   A. Decreased circulatory and respiratory function
      1.  Monitor vital signs and neurologic reflex responses
      2.  Suction as necessary
      3.  Monitor the need for cardiopulmonary resuscitation

   B. Impending withdrawal
      1.  Assess the current stage of withdrawal
      2.  Administer medications, as ordered
      3.  Approach the client calmly; avoid touching the client
      4.  Limit visitors

   C. Potential for self-injury
      1.  Restrain the client as needed
      2.  Remove harmful objects
      3.  Monitor suicidal behavior

   D. Panic and flashback reactions
      1.  Remain with the client
      2.  Encourage expression of feelings
      3.  Provide reassurance by orienting the client to reality
      4.  Do not support delusions or hallucinations

   E. Poor nutritional status
      1.  Administer skin care
      2.  Record fluid and nutritional intake and output
      3.  Administer I.V. solutions when prescribed
      4.  Provide small, frequent feedings

## XV. Nursing care problems and interventions in drug rehabilitation

   A. Denial of the illness
      1.  Focus on the problem of substance abuse

2. Avoid the client's attempts to focus only on external problems
3. Identify the projection of blame or defensiveness
4. Avoid discussions of unanswerable questions

B. Lack of knowledge about consequences of drug use
   1. Provide factual information
   2. Dispel myths

C. Avoidance of responsibility
   1. Encourage the client to identify behaviors that cause difficulties
   2. Do not allow the client to rationalize or to blame others
   3. Refocus on the client's problems
   4. Encourage others to provide feedback
   5. Positively reinforce expressions of feelings and insights
   6. Encourage verbal expression of anger and depression
   7. Provide a structured environment
   8. Prepare the client for a change in life-style
   9. Discuss alternative methods of dealing with stress

D. Discharge planning
   1. Identify support systems
   2. Encourage compliance with treatment
   3. Explore goals for discharge

# XVI. Additional treatments for rehabilitation stages of substance abuse

A. Individual therapy

B. Social support systems
   1. Family counseling
   2. Self-help groups (such as Alcoholics Anonymous and Synanon)
   3. Halfway houses
   4. Employee assistance programs

C. Group therapy

D. BEHAVIOR MODIFICATION

E. Pharmacology
   1. Antabuse
   2. Methadone maintenance

# XVII. Evaluation

A. Base the evaluation on realistic expectations

B. Reevaluate at regular intervals

C. Analyze behavioral outcomes

D. Complete a self-evaluation

## Points to remember

Any drug can be misused.

Substance abuse is a behavioral pattern that involves all aspects of the client's functioning.

Substance abuse poses a major health problem in the United States.

No simple cause of substance abuse has been identified or accepted.

In the acute stage of drug intoxication, maintaining the client's physical well-being takes priority.

## Glossary

The following terms are defined in Appendix A, page 142.

addiction

behavior modification

psychological dependence

tolerance

withdrawal syndrome

## Study questions

To evaluate your understanding of this chapter, answer the following questions in the space provided; then compare your responses with the correct answers in Appendix B, pages 153 and 154.

1. Which behaviors might a nurse observe in a substance abuser? _____

_____

_____

2. What are three predisposing psychological factors associated with substance abuse? _____

_____

3. Which behaviors are associated with each phase of alcoholism? _____

_____

4. How can the nurse intervene during alcohol withdrawal? _____

_____

5. What are three problems that the nurse may have to confront during the rehabilitative stage of alcoholism? _____

_____

6. If a client is suspected of inhalant abuse, which behaviors might be exhibited? _____

_____

7. Which problems should a nurse anticipate during a client's acute drug reaction? _____

_____

8. How should a nurse handle a client's denial during drug rehabilitation?

_____

_____

## CHAPTER 13

# Anger

**Learning objectives**

Check off the following items once you've mastered them:

☐ Identify the seven positive functions of anger.

☐ Describe physical, emotional, intellectual, social, and spiritual responses that indicate anger.

☐ Formulate appropriate nursing diagnoses for clients experiencing anger.

☐ List at least eight interventions a nurse could use in dealing with an angry client.

☐ Evaluate nursing interventions for clients experiencing anger.

# I. General characteristics of anger

    A. Serves as a natural adaptation to disruption

    B. Is characterized by tension

    C. Occurs in response to anxiety from a perceived threat

    D. Ranges from mild annoyance to rage or fury

    E. Is related to a fear of rejection

# II. Functional anger

    A. Energizes behavior to avoid anxiety

    B. Characterizes a healthy relationship

    C. Can project a positive self-concept

    D. Serves as an ego defense; more effective than anxiety

    E. Gives the person a sense of control

    F. Indicates a need for more effective coping behaviors

    G. Provides immediate relief

# III. Dysfunctional anger

    A. Arises when early conflicts are reenacted

    B. Becomes a source of tension

    C. Is cyclical, stemming from or resulting in:
        1. Unresolved anxiety and anger
        2. Offensive behaviors
        3. Powerlessness in others
        4. Angry response or rejection by others

# IV. Modes of expression

    A. External
        1. Constructive criticism
        2. AGGRESSION

    B. Internal
        1. Nonassertiveness
        2. Self-destruction

    C. Direct

    D. Indirect
        1. Passivity
        2. Manipulation
        3. Acting-out behavior

E. Displaced onto safe objects

## V. Precipitating stressors

A. Individualized

B. External or internal threatening event

## VI. Assessment

A. Physical responses associated with anger (resulting from action of the autonomic nervous system in response to epinephrine secretion)
   1. Increased blood pressure
   2. Tachycardia
   3. Altered blood composition
   4. Increased salivation
   5. Nausea
   6. Increased hydrochloric acid secretion
   7. Decreased gastric peristalsis
   8. Increased alertness and muscle tension
   9. Accelerated reflexes
   10. Increased urination
   11. Dilated pupils
   12. Flushed face
   13. Sweating

B. Emotional responses associated with anger
   1. Discomfort
   2. Powerlessness
   3. Annoyance
   4. Frustration
   5. Resentment
   6. Belligerence
   7. Rage
   8. Humiliation
   9. Defensiveness
   10. Inadequacy
   11. Depression
   12. HOSTILITY
   13. Guilt
   14. Acting-out behavior

C. Intellectual responses associated with anger
   1. Sarcasm
   2. Argumentativeness
   3. Fault finding
   4. Domination
   5. Belittling

6. Scolding
7. Blaming
8. Forgetfulness
9. Repetitive thoughts
10. RUMINATION
11. Projection
12. Ridicule

D. Social responses associated with anger
1. Withdrawal
2. Alienation
3. Rejection
4. Teasing
5. Humor
6. Violence
7. Poor self-concept
8. Demand making
9. Intimidation
10. Overactivity
11. Hypersensitivity
12. Substance abuse

E. Spiritual responses associated with anger
1. Omnipotence
2. Self-righteousness
3. Self-doubt
4. Demoralization
5. Sinfulness
6. Blocked creativity

## VII. Diagnoses

A. *DSM-III-R* medical diagnoses
1. Oppositional disorder
2. Conduct disorder
3. Delusional (paranoid) disorder
4. Organic personality syndrome (explosive type)

B. Primary NANDA diagnostic categories
1. Potential for violence directed at others
2. Ineffective individual coping

C. Secondary NANDA diagnostic categories
1. Anxiety
2. Impaired verbal communication
3. Dysfunctional grieving
4. Potential for injury
5. Powerlessness

6.  Self-esteem disturbance
7.  Social isolation

## VIII. Nursing care goals

A. Establish hierarchy of behaviors

B. Reinforce mastery and self-control

## IX. Nursing interventions

A. Provide constructive outlets, protection, and control

B. Remain with the client, and do not become defensive

C. Set and enforce appropriate limits

D. Reduce sources of anxiety

E. Acknowledge the client's anger, and help the client recognize those feelings

F. Encourage the client to describe angry feelings and to explore reasons for the anger

G. Clarify misunderstandings

H. Communicate that anger is acceptable

I.  Help the client use assertive behaviors

J.  Enhance the client's self-esteem

K. Monitor personal anxiety level

L. Prevent violence

## X. Evaluation

A. Evaluate the client's progress in controlling anger, noting these factors:
1.  Behavioral changes
2.  Subjective responses of the client
3.  Appropriateness of expressions of anger
4.  Use of assertive behaviors
5.  Successful problem solving

B. Complete a nursing self-assessment of nontherapeutic responses
1.  Defensiveness
2.  Retaliation
3.  Condescension
4.  Avoidance

## Points to remember

Anger is a natural response to feelings of inadequacy and may be expressed overtly or covertly, externally or internally.

Anger is experienced on a continuum from mild annoyance to intense rage.

Anger serves many positive functions.

Nurses should be aware of their own feelings and responses when intervening with the angry client.

## Glossary

The following terms are defined in Appendix A, page 142.

aggression

hostility

rumination

## Study questions

To evaluate your understanding of this chapter, answer the following questions in the space provided; then compare your responses to the correct answers in Appendix B, page 154.

1. How does functional anger differ from dysfunctional anger? _____

_____

_____

2. In which two forms can anger be expressed externally? _____

_____

3. Which are the two nursing care goals for a client experiencing anger?

_____

_____

4. Which factors would the nurse consider when evaluating a client's response to nursing interventions for anger? _____

_____

## CHAPTER 14

# Assaultive Behavior

## Learning objectives

Check off the following items once you've mastered them:

☐ Compare and contrast aggression and violence.

☐ Name at least six factors that increase one's potential for violence.

☐ Formulate appropriate nursing diagnoses for clients experiencing aggressive behavior and for those who are victims of sexual assault.

☐ Develop nursing care plans for intervening in verbally and physically aggressive behavior.

☐ Describe three nursing interventions for clients who have been sexually assaulted.

# I. Characteristics of aggression

A. A natural drive
   1. Is destructive when uncontrolled
   2. Evokes the defensive response
   3. Can be instrumental or hostile
   4. Can be direct or indirect

B. A precursor of violence

# II. Theories of aggression

A. Psychoanalytic theory
   1. AGGRESSION is instinctual
   2. The aggressor attempts to master personal inferiority

B. Drive theory (frustration-aggression theory)
   1. Frustration occurs when goal achievement is blocked, which leads to anger, anxiety, and aggression
   2. This innate response can be inhibited

C. Social learning theory
   1. Aggression is a learned behavior
   2. The social environment instigates and reinforces aggression

D. Need theory
   1. Aggression is a method of communicating a need
   2. When a need cannot be met through constructive behavior, aggression (destructive behavior) is used

E. Stress adaptation theory
   1. Any activity requiring a response generates stress
   2. Stress carries the potential for violence

F. Biochemical theory
   1. The limbic system regulates aggressive behavior
   2. A lesion of the hypothalamus and amygdala increases or decreases aggressive behavior
   3. Release of norepinephrine by the adrenal medulla directly influences aggressive behavior
   4. Increased blood levels of testosterone in males correlate with increased aggressiveness
   5. Decreased progesterone blood levels in females correlate with increased hostility

# III. VIOLENCE

A. Characteristics
   1. Carries physical, emotional, or moral force
   2. Poses a threat to others and arouses their fears

      3. Creates anxiety in victims
      4. Is displayed deliberately or follows a loss of control over aggressive impulses

B. Precipitating factors
      1. Psychotic conditions and impaired thought processes
      2. Organic conditions
      3. Depression
      4. Disorders of impulse control; antisocial behavior
      5. Ineffective coping skills
      6. Dysfunctional family systems
      7. Disturbed roles within the family system
      8. Disturbed marital relationships
      9. Violent expressions of anger

C. Assessment: Behavioral cues
      1. Change in usual behavior
      2. Glaring
      3. Restlessness
      4. Rigid posture
      5. Clenched hands
      6. Ingestion of alcohol or drugs
      7. Overt, aggressive actions
      8. Physical withdrawal
      9. Noncompliance
    10. Overreaction
    11. Hostile threats
    12. Talk of past violent acts
    13. Inability to express feelings
    14. Repetitive demands and complaints
    15. Argumentativeness
    16. Profanity
    17. Abusive belittling
    18. Disorientation
    19. Inability to focus attention
    20. Hallucinations or delusions
    21. Paranoid ideas or suspicions
    22. Somatic complaint or preoccupation

D. Diagnoses
      1. *DSM-III-R* medical diagnoses
         a. Personality disorder
         b. Organic mental disorder
         c. Intermittent explosive disorder
         d. Isolated explosive disorder
         e. Impulse control disorder (not otherwise specified)
         f. Organic personality disorder

      g. Delusional disorders

  2. Primary NANDA diagnostic categories

      a. Ineffective individual coping

      b. Potential for self-directed violence

      c. Potential for violence directed at others

      d. Anxiety

E. Nursing care goals

  1. Prevent further loss of control in a potentially violent client

  2. Restore a violent client's self-control

F. Nursing interventions

  1. For a potentially violent client

      a. Be aware of precursive signs

      b. Ask other clients or visitors to leave the area

      c. Maintain a reasonable physical distance from the client

      d. Explain to the client all actions that the staff will carry out

      e. Offer reassurance of safety

      f. Remove objects that could be used destructively

      g. Seek assistance from other health care personnel, if needed

      h. Provide sedation, if required and prescribed

      i. Help the client distinguish among thoughts, feelings, and behaviors

      j. Explore alternative behaviors

      k. Encourage the client to consider the consequences of violent behavior

      l. Set firm limits

  2. For a verbally aggressive client

      a. Remain with the client

      b. Do not become angry or defensive

      c. Be aware of personal anxiety level

      d. Provide consistent expectations and guidelines for the client's self-control

      e. Acknowledge the client's anger, and state that anger is an acceptable feeling

      f. Explore the precipitating threat or frustration

      g. Promote insight into the need for control

  3. For a physically aggressive client

      a. Take precautions to ensure personal safety; do not attempt to handle the client alone

      b. Approach the client calmly and firmly

      c. Use short, concise statements

      d. Inform the client of what is expected

      e. Provide medication

      f. Arrange for SECLUSION of the client

G. Evaluation

  1. Meet with staff members to review any violent behavior of a client

2. Dissipate staff anxiety
3. Review outcome criteria
4. Discuss with the client ways to prevent violent behavior
5. Acknowledge improvements in the client's ability to express anger constructively

# IV. Sexual assault

A. Characteristics
1. Comprises verbal assaults, threats, intimidation, and physical force without the victim's consent
2. Constitutes a traumatic event that serves as a precursor of crisis

B. Incidence
1. Lack of accurate information on prevalence because assault victims typically are reluctant to report the assault
2. Increase in report of sexual abuse of children, although experts say that most cases still go unreported

D. Motivations for sexual assault
1. An act of aggression (it is *not* a sexual act)
2. A means of gaining control
3. A desire to humiliate, defile, or dominate the victim

E. Reactions of rape victims
1. Panic during the attack
2. Humiliation, confusion, fear, and rage after the attack
3. Long-term emotional effects (persist for several years)
   a. Victimization and vulnerability
   b. Degradation
   c. Shame
   d. Guilt
   e. Self-blame
   f. Wish for revenge

F. Assessment
1. Related to the victim
   a. Emotional and mental assessment
   b. Physical assessment
   c. History of the assault
   d. Reaction to the assault
   e. Meaning of the assault for the victim
   f. Potential help-seeking behaviors
2. Related to the nurse
   a. Personal response
   b. Societal biases
   c. Myths
   d. Degree of self-awareness

3. Related to the family
   a. Support systems
   b. Response of others to the victim
4. Related to the community
   a. Police
   b. Rape crisis center or other community groups

G. Diagnoses
   1. *DSM-III-R* medical diagnosis: Post-traumatic stress disorder
   2. NANDA diagnostic category: Rape trauma syndrome

H. Nursing care goals
   1. Restore the client's emotional control and previous functioning
   2. Help the client rediscover self-respect and dignity

I. Nursing interventions
   1. Follow institutional protocols for notifying the police and collecting evidence of sexual assault
      a. Record the date, the time, and the officer's name
      b. Collect evidence (clothing, fingernail scrapings, semen) in the presence of a witness, label the evidence carefully, and document findings
   2. Perform a thorough assessment and physical examination
      a. Observe the client's general appearance; measure and record vital signs
      b. Obtain a medical history, including the rape
      c. Note signs of vaginal or anal bleeding, bruises, lacerations, and redness; measure the size and note the location of injuries
      d. Obtain vaginal swabs and smears
      e. Advise the client of a 6-week follow-up examination to rule out sexually transmitted diseases
      f. Document findings
   3. Take steps to support the client emotionally
      a. Pursue CRISIS INTERVENTION when warranted, such as in rape trauma syndrome
      b. Provide a private, quiet environment where the client can feel safe and think clearly
      c. Encourage the client to discuss the assault, if able
      d. Initially, focus on the client's immediate feelings (such as guilt, shame, or ambivalence); then discuss other issues, such as the client's options, possible legal procedures, and counseling
      e. Refer the client for continuing counseling, if desired

J. Treatment modalities
   1. Crisis intervention
   2. Hospital emergency departments
   3. Individual counseling
   4. Behavior modification

    5.  Social support systems
    6.  Assertiveness training
    7.  Victim group sessions
    8.  Family sessions
    9.  Spiritual counseling

K. Evaluation
    1.  Note the client's identification of needs
    2.  Apply outcome criteria

## Points to remember

Violence and assaultive behavior are unhealthy, destructive expressions of aggressive drive.

Intervention with a violent client should focus on immediate control and safety.

Sexual assault is an act of aggression.

Nursing interventions for victims of sexual assault vary and must be individualized to meet the client's needs.

## Glossary

The following terms are defined in Appendix A, page 142.

aggression

crisis intervention

seclusion

violence

## Study questions

To evaluate your understanding of this chapter, answer the following questions in the space provided; then compare your responses to the correct answers in Appendix B, page 155.

1. What are the characteristics of violence? _____

_____

2. How should a nurse intervene with a physically aggressive client? _____

_____

_____

3. What are three motivations for sexual assault? _____

_____

4. What should the nurse do with evidence collected in a sexual assault case?

_____

_____

## CHAPTER 15

# Family Abuse and Violence

## Learning objectives

Check off the following items once you've mastered them:

☐ Differentiate between violence and abuse.

☐ Identify five characteristics of a violent family system.

☐ Formulate individualized nursing diagnoses for offenders and victims.

☐ Describe nursing interventions that consider the needs of each family member.

## I. Definitions

A. *Abuse:* acts of misuse, exploitation, or deceit intended to injure, damage, maltreat, or corrupt

B. *Violence:* exertion of extreme force or destructive action to injure or harm

C. *Family violence:* physical, psychological, sexual, material, or social violation or exploitation of a person by a family member

## II. Categories of family violence

A. Physical abuse
1. Slapping, kicking, or punching
2. Hitting or whipping with a blunt instrument
3. Pulling hair
4. Inflicting burns
5. Throwing an individual
6. Choking or gagging
7. Tying to a bed, chair, or crib
8. Locking in a closet or room for an extended period
9. Attempting to drown or hang

B. Neglect
1. Failure to provide food, bed, shelter, clothing, health care, or sensory stimulation or to meet hygiene needs
2. Inability or refusal to protect against accidents or otherwise ensure safety

C. Psychological unavailability
1. Ignorance of an individual's needs
2. Failure to provide sufficient affection or warmth
3. Inability to appreciate acomplishment or competence
4. Failure to respect privacy, preferences, or opinions
5. Unwillingness to share pleasant experiences or social events

D. Verbal hostility
1. Name calling
2. Use of obscenities
3. Severe criticism
4. Use of humiliation and shame
5. Threats

E. Sexual abuse
1. Rape
2. Sodomy
3. INCEST
4. EXHIBITIONISM (sometimes accompanied by masturbation)

## III. Epidemiology of family violence

A. Spouse abuse
1. Women are usually the victims; wife abuse is the most common cause of trauma in women
2. The problem spans all socioeconomic classes
3. 15% to 20% of homicides involve spouse abuse

B. Child abuse
1. Few reliable statistics exist
2. The problem spans all socioeconomic classes

C. Elder abuse
1. An estimated 10% of elderly adults are abused
2. The abuser is typically the elderly person's adult child
3. Elder abuse also occurs in institutions, such as nursing homes

## IV. Etiologic theories

A. Psychodynamic theory
1. Deprivation of nurturance in childhood
2. Victim of physical or sexual abuse as a child
3. Antisocial behavior
4. Mental illness

B. Social learning theory
1. Lack of healthy role models for parenting and problem solving
2. A learned response; typically evident in many generations of the same family

C. Environmental stress theory
1. Stress (such as from unemployment or poverty) that triggers abuse
2. Societal factors that promote and maintain violent expression
3. Inequity between stronger and weaker persons
4. Socialization that teaches women and children to be subservient

D. Family systems theory
1. Faulty structure in family system
2. Inability of family members to define themselves as individuals apart from the family
3. Conflict within the family system

## V. Assessment

A. Characteristics of the violent family system
1. Closed boundaries
2. Painful and desperate mood

   3. Competition for affection, caring, attention, and nurturance
   4. Inability of family members to define themselves as individuals apart from the family
   5. Inability to trust others
   6. Conflict within the family system
   7. Lack of impulse control and self-discipline
   8. Reduced capacity to delay gratification
   9. Focus on the present
  10. Inadequate task performance
  11. Mixed or double messages in communications
  12. Faulty perception of reality
  13. Imbalanced power ratio (one member has control over other members)
  14. Stereotyping of roles

B. Characteristics of offenders and victims
  1. Offender
    a. Exhibits cyclical behavior
    b. Is immature and lacks self-control
    c. Displays insecurity
    d. Is dominant, rigid, and moralistic
    e. Shows aggressiveness
    f. Needs immediate gratification
    g. Lacks guilt
    h. Has symbiotic personality and poor interpersonal relationships
    i. Exhibits substance abuse
  2. Abusing parent
    a. Is depressed
    b. Has unrealistic expectations of the child (as if the child were much older)
    c. Looks to children as a source of reassurance while projecting own problems onto the children
    d. Lacks confidence in parenting abilities, so feels children are the source of troubles
    e. Has hypochondriacal complaints
    f. Has a history of having been abused
  3. Spouse victim
    a. Displays ambivalence or fear
    b. Has low self-esteem, so feels responsible for provoking anger
    c. Rationalizes the abuse
    d. Is socially isolated
  4. Child victim
    a. Runs away from home
    b. Displays age-inappropriate sexual behavior
    c. Is one whose age, sex, physical appearance, or personality may trigger conflict for the parent
    d. Shows ambivalence, depression, anxiety, fear

   5. Elderly victim
      a. Is demanding and may act helpless or hopeless before the abuse
      b. May be belligerent and aggressive before the abuse

C. Physical symptoms
   1. Bruises
   2. Lacerations
   3. Broken bones
   4. Symptoms of anxiety and stress
   5. Chronic fatigue
   6. Old scars and bruises
   7. Bite marks
   8. Burns
   9. Blackened eyes
   10. Retarded growth or development
   11. Poor hygiene

D. Behavioral cues
   1. General
      a. Inconsistent or irrational account of causes of injuries
      b. Significant time lapse between injury and treatment
      c. Family member's refusal to permit diagnostic tests; hasty exit from
         the examination room
      d. Unwillingness of significant other to comfort the victim
   2. Cues related to all victims
      a. Withdrawal or extreme aggression
      b. Tendency to startle easily
      c. Disturbed sleep patterns
      d. Evasive comments about injury
      e. Avoidance of eye contact
      f. Vacant or frozen stare
      g. Chronic lateness or truancy from job or school
      h. Delinquent behavior
      i. Apology for seeking treatment
   3. Cues related to child victims
      a. Wariness of adults
      b. Rapid adaptation to hospital unit
      c. Unwillingness to turn to family member or parents for support
      d. Abnormal eating or drinking habits
      e. Excessive or absent crying
      f. Extreme fear of or total lack of respect for authority figures

## VI. Diagnoses

A. *DSM-III-R* medical diagnoses: none

B. Primary NANDA diagnostic categories
   1. Ineffective individual coping

    2. Ineffective family coping: compromised
    3. Ineffective family coping: disabled
    4. Family coping: potential for growth

C. Secondary NANDA diagnostic categories
    1. Anxiety
    2. Impaired communication
    3. Alterations in family process
    4. Fear
    5. Potential for injury
    6. Knowledge deficit
    7. Alterations in parenting
    8. Post-trauma response
    9. Impaired social interaction
   10. Social isolation
   11. Potential for violence

## VII. Nursing care goals

A. Individualize goals and interventions according to the form and type of violence

B. Help the family function at a healthier level

C. Offer individualized treatment to the client and family

D. Maintain self-awareness during intervention

## VIII. Nursing interventions

A. Report abuse to authorities

B. Ensure the client's safety

C. Refer the client and family to appropriate resources

D. Arrange for a medical examination

E. Collect evidence (such as the location and extent of injuries)

F. Offer anticipatory guidance and counseling

G. Explain legal procedures

H. Separate the victim from the offender

## IX. Treatment modalities

A. CRISIS INTERVENTION

B. Individual counseling

    C. Support groups

    D. Family therapy

    E. Community support services

## X. Evaluation

    A. Complete a nursing self-assessment

    B. Determine the effectiveness of nursing interventions in meeting the client's physical care needs

    C. Ensure that the client's medical record is complete and accurate

## Points to remember

Family abuse and violence span all socioeconomic classes.

Violence is commonly a learned behavior that persists in many generations of the same family.

Self-awareness by the nurse is essential for intervention.

Nursing goals and interventions must be individualized according to the form and type of family violence encountered.

## Glossary

The following terms are defined in Appendix A, page 142.

crisis intervention

exhibitionism

incest

## Study questions

To evaluate your understanding of this chapter, answer the following questions in the space provided; then compare your responses to the correct answers in Appendix B, page 155.

1. What is abuse? _____

_____

2. What are the five categories of family violence? _____

_____

3. What are the major characteristics of a violent family system? _____

_____

4. Which behavioral clues should a nurse look for when assessing a possible victim of child abuse? _____

_____

5. What is an essential part of the nursing care plan for a client experiencing family abuse and violence? _____

_____

# Treatment Modalities and the Role of the Psychiatric Nurse

## Learning objectives

Check off the following items once you've mastered them:

☐ Describe six treatment modalities used with psychiatric clients.

☐ Discuss assumptions underlying crisis intervention, therapeutic environment, group approaches, family therapy, individual psychotherapy, and biological therapy.

☐ Identify at least six curative factors for individual and group approaches.

☐ Compare and contrast strategies of intervention in various treatment approaches.

☐ Discuss the role of the nurse in each of the treatment modalities.

## I. CRISIS INTERVENTION

A. Assumptions
   1. Crisis is a temporary state that occurs when stress overwhelms an individual's usual coping mechanisms
   2. Crisis is self-limiting, typically resolving within 6 weeks
   3. Crisis intervention is an appropriate action for all nurses in all settings

B. Predisposing factors
   1. Disastrous event
   2. Threatened loss of a basic gratification
   3. Failure to cope with stress
   4. Perceived absence of situational support

C. Phases
   1. Anxiety in response to a perceived threat or event
   2. Disorganization with increased general anxiety
   3. State of emergency with resolution or defeat
   4. Breaking point

D. Types
   1. Developmental-maturational crisis
   2. Situational crisis
   3. Victim crises

E. Characteristics of intervention
   1. Increases the likelihood that a crisis will be positively resolved
   2. Offers immediate help and reestablishes equilibrium
   3. Restores the client's precrisis level of functioning
   4. Teaches the client new ways of problem solving

F. Phases of intervention
   1. Assess the nature of the crisis, its effect on the client, and the client's coping mechanisms and support systems
   2. Begin planning: formulate dynamics, explore options, designate steps to arrive at solutions
   3. Intervene through environmental manipulation, general support, or a generic or individual approach
      a. Environmental manipulation provides direct situational support or removes stress (such as arranging for someone to stay with the client)
      b. General support reassures the client that the health care professional understands and will help the client (for example, by providing empathy)
      c. A generic approach uses a standard intervention for all individuals faced with the same crisis
      d. An individual approach uses interventions tailored to a particular client
   4. Evaluate whether the crisis has been positively resolved

G. Techniques of intervention
   1. Take an active, focal, and exploratory approach
   2. Maintain the client's present orientation
   3. Guide intervention through its phases
   4. Encourage expression of feelings and an awareness of the links among events, current feelings, and behavior
   5. Persuade the client to view the therapist as a helper
   6. Promote and reinforce adaptive behavior
   7. Do not attack the client's defenses
   8. Increase the client's self-esteem
   9. Explore solutions to the problem causing the crisis

H. Alternative strategies
   1. Telephone crisis counseling
   2. Emergency room crisis counseling
   3. Home visits
   4. Family crisis counseling
   5. Crisis group therapy

I. Role of the nurse
   1. Assess the crisis
   2. Offer individual crisis therapy
   3. Organize crisis groups
   4. Participate in disaster work
   5. Use preventive intervention
   6. Provide client education

## II. Therapeutic environment

A. Assumptions
   1. Scientific manipulation of the environment can change the client's personality
   2. Clients have strengths as well as conflict-free portions of their personalities, so they can constructively influence treatment
   3. Successful treatment depends on therapeutic staff involvement at all levels
   4. Human behavior can change in response to physical, interpersonal, and cultural environments

B. Characteristics of intervention
   1. Focuses on a client's interaction with the environment
   2. Creates an atmosphere in which the client can develop appropriate responses to individuals and situations
   3. Is deliberately planned and structured to modify maladaptive responses
   4. Promotes positive insights and responses

C. Treatment modalities
1. MILIEU THERAPY
2. Therapeutic community
3. Community meeting
4. Client-team meeting
5. Therapeutic recreation
6. Occupational therapy
7. Music and art therapy
8. Horticulture therapy
9. Social work therapy

D. Techniques
1. Encourage, develop, and maintain communication between staff and client
2. Hold weekly staff meetings
3. Set limits on and establish external controls over unacceptable behaviors
4. Foster the client's psychosocial skills
5. Assess and implement individual treatment modalities
6. Create a homelike atmosphere
7. Focus treatment on action and problem solving

E. Role of the nurse
1. Act as a role model primarily in inpatient settings
2. Facilitate and oversee implementation of interventions
3. Structure the client's environment

## III. Group approaches

A. Assumptions
1. Human beings are social animals that desire interaction with others
2. Group therapy can alleviate intrapsychic distress or modify personality traits
3. Therapeutic groups focus on interpersonal, cognitive, or behavioral changes
4. Group dynamics can help modify behavior
5. Groups offer a safe environment for sharing emotional experiences

B. Stages of group development
1. Initial: conflict issues are dependency and authority
2. Middle: conflict issues are intimacy, cooperation, and productivity
3. Final: conflict issues are disengagement and dissolution

C. Leadership styles
1. Democratic: encourages all members to participate in decision making
2. Autocratic: maintains control over decision making
3. Laissez-faire: relinquishes all control over decision making and provides little, if any, guidance or support

D. Membership roles in groups
   1. Task roles: administrative and goal-oriented
   2. Maintenance roles: enhance group interaction
   3. Egocentric roles: express individual emotional needs

E. Curative factors in groups
   1. Guidance
   2. Altruism
   3. Cohesion
   4. Catharsis
   5. Identification
   6. Family reenactment
   7. Interpersonal learning: input
   8. Interpersonal learning: output
   9. Universality
   10. Insight
   11. Instillation of hope
   12. EXISTENTIALISM

F. Types of group leadership
   1. Single therapist
   2. Co-therapist
   3. Leaderless

G. Types of group therapies
   1. Self-help groups
   2. Psychotherapeutic groups
   3. PSYCHODRAMA
   4. Multiple-family group therapy

H. Types of therapeutic groups
   1. Self-help groups
   2. Remotivation and reeducation groups
   3. Client-government groups
   4. Activity therapy groups
   5. Client teaching-education groups

I. Role of the nurse in group approaches
   1. Group therapy must be conducted by a clinical specialist with a master's degree and a history of supervised clinical practice with groups
   2. Therapeutic groups can be conducted by all nurses in all settings

## IV. Family therapy

A. Assumptions
   1. Dysfunction in a client usually originates in the family
   2. The family is the client, and the focus is on family interaction
   3. The goal is to enable each family member to function independently

B. Models
1. Structural therapy
2. Strategic therapy

C. Techniques and strategies
1. Co-therapy
2. Single therapist
3. Network therapy
4. Operational mourning
5. Sculpting
6. Role playing
7. Paradoxical injunction
8. Home visits

D. Role of the nurse
1. A generalist nurse sees clients in a family context, recognizes functional and dysfunctional behavior patterns, then makes referrals
2. A clinical specialist works as a family therapist and consultant

# V. Individual psychotherapy

A. Assumptions
1. Therapy uses interpersonal relationships to effect positive changes in the client's psychological well-being
2. The need for help is typically expressed as a symptom
3. The client is anxious

B. Curative factors common to all theoretical approaches
1. Common goal linking the therapist and the client
2. Mobilization of the client's hope
3. Anticipatory guidance
4. Verbal communications
5. Universality
6. Emotional arousal
7. Provision of new information
8. Insight into the problem's origin
9. Development of new problem-solving skills
10. Social learning experiences (such as new techniques for communicating with others)
11. Imitative behavior
12. Intense, confiding relationship

C. Types
1. Crisis intervention
2. Time-limited therapy
3. Supportive therapy
4. Long-term therapy
5. Psychodynamic therapy

6. Cognitive therapy

D. Role of the nurse
1. A clinical specialist acts as a psychotherapist in therapy
2. A generalist nurse acts as a supportive therapist by counseling and by maintaining the nurse-client relationship

## VI. Biological therapies

A. Assumptions
1. Biological therapies follow a medical model
2. They focus on symptoms, diagnoses, and prognoses

B. Types of biological treatments
1. Psychotropic medications
2. Electroconvulsive therapy
3. Narcotherapy
4. PSYCHOSURGERY
5. Insulin coma treatment
6. Niacin therapy
7. Electrosleep therapy
8. Nonconvulsive electrical stimulation therapy
9. Hemodialysis

C. Role of the nurse
1. Function as a client advocate
2. Educate the client
3. Administer medications
4. Support the client before, during, and after treatment
5. Observe the client for side effects

## Points to remember

Nurses must understand various treatment modalities to coordinate total care.

The role of the nurse varies with each treatment modality.

A nurse must act only in roles for which he or she is educationally and clinically prepared.

The nurse's primary role is that of client advocate.

## Glossary

The following terms are defined in Appendix A, page 142.

crisis intervention                    psychodrama

existentialism                         psychosurgery

milieu therapy

## Study questions

To evaluate your understanding of this chapter, answer the following questions in the space provided; then compare your responses with the correct answers in Appendix B, pages 155 and 156.

1. What is a crisis? How long does it usually last?_____

_____

2. What are the major characteristics of crisis intervention? _____

_____

3. What is the nurse's role in a therapeutic environment? _____

_____

4. What are the three membership roles assumed in a group? _____

_____

5. What is the focus of family therapy? _____

_____

6. What are the roles of the clinical nurse specialist and the nurse generalist in individual psychotherapy? _____

_____

7. What is the focus of biological therapies? _____

_____

# Appendices

## A: Glossary

**Adaptation** — organism's adjustment to its environment

**Addiction** — compulsive use of a chemical substance that contributes to physical or psychological dependence

**Affect** — outward manifestation of emotions

**Aggression** — mental drive that can lead to constructive or destructive activities

**Alienation** — withdrawal or detachment from society

**Anticipatory guidance** — information and advice given to clients for future therapeutic purposes

**Attitudinal restructuring** — alteration of a position taken on an issue

**Autistic thinking** — ideas that have private meaning to the individual

**Autogenic training** — therapy that attempts to establish functional harmony by using natural forces in the brain

**Aversion therapy** — application of a painful stimulus to promote avoidance of unacceptable behavior

**Behavior modification** — method of reeducation based on Pavlovian conditioning principles

**Biofeedback** — use of electrodes and tonal pitch to reduce tension

**Body image** — internalized impressions and attitudes about one's physical self

**Clang association** — speech pattern characterized by rhyming

**Community mental health** — treatment philosophy advocating a comprehensive range of mental health services available to all community members

**Consensual validation** — reinforcement of meanings and interpretations by evidence and corroboration from others

**Conversion disorder**—somatoform disorder characterized by psychogenic disturbances of motor or sensory activity

**Coping mechanisms**—techniques used to protect oneself from the effects of anxiety

**Counter-conditioning**—replacement of a learned response with a less disruptive one

**Crisis intervention**—short-term therapy intended to reestablish a level of functioning equal to or better than the precrisis level

**Defense mechanisms**—unconscious coping mechanisms that a person uses to prevent awareness of anxiety or to mask feelings of inadequacy or worthlessness

**Degenerative dementia**—irreversible deterioration of mental capacities

**Delusions**—false, fixed beliefs not validated by reality and firmly held despite contradictory information

**Depersonalization**—feelings of estrangement and separateness from oneself

**Depression**—psychological state characterized by dejection, lowered self-esteem, hopelessness, helplessness, indecision, and rumination

**Desensitization**—gradual exposure to a predetermined stress-producing stimulus on a continuum from least to most severe

**Dichotomous thinking**—categorization of events, objects, or ideas into two, usually opposing, parts

**Echolalia**—purposeless repetition of a word or phrase just spoken by someone else

**Ego-dystonic behaviors**—behaviors that disrupt one's identity or sense of self

**Ego-syntonic behaviors**—behaviors that are compatible with one's identity or sense of self

**Empathy**—ability to understand the feelings of others and to respond sensitively

**Encounter group therapy**—therapy that focuses on the reaction of members to events in the group

**Exhibitionism** — sexual gratification obtained through public exposure of the genitals

**Existentialism** — school of philosophical thought that focuses on the present and presumes that a person finds meaning in life through experiences

**Feedback** — process by which functioning is monitored, corrected (if inappropriate), and maintained (if appropriate)

**Fight-or-flight response** — sympathetic nervous system response to anxiety in which an individual deals with a stressful situation or avoids it

**Free association** — psychoanalytic technique in which the client articulates all thoughts

**Gestalt therapy** — therapy that focuses on enhancement of self-awareness

**Grieving** — subjective response to the loss of a highly valued person or object

**Guided imagery** — therapy that controls anxiety by helping the client visualize successful coping with a stressful event

**Holistic** — viewing a human being as a unified biologic, psychological, and social organism

**Hostility** — anger and resentment characterized by destructive behavior

**Hypochondriasis** — depression marked by a persistent fear or belief that one has a serious illness

**Id** — mental structure in psychoanalytic theory that represents unconscious drives and impulses

**Identity** — sense of selfhood that sustains an integrated personality structure

**Incest** — sexual relationship between persons who are biologically related

**Magical thinking** — belief that one's thoughts or wishes can control other people or events

**Mania** — psychological state characterized by an elevated or expansive mood

**Milieu** — social and cultural aspects of the treatment setting that can reduce behavioral disturbances

**Milieu therapy** — manipulation of a client's sociocultural environment to reduce behavioral disturbances

**Mutism**—lack of speech

**Neologism**—invented word understood only by the inventor

**Neurotic behavior**—dysfunctional behavior characterized by anxiety without reality distortion

**Operant conditioning**—behavior modification through systematic manipulation of antecedents and consequences

**Perception**—response of sensory receptors to external stimuli that involves both cognitive and emotional knowledge

**Primary prevention**—actions taken to reduce the incidence of disease

**Projection**—attribution of blame or responsibility for one's acts and feelings to other people

**Psychodrama**—structured, directed dramatization of a client's personal, emotional, and interactional problems

**Psychogenic fugue**—maladaptive response to a problem with self-concept in which the client assumes a new identity after sudden, unexpected travel away from home or work

**Psychogenic pain**—pain originating in the mind

**Psychological dependence**—subjective feeling that a certain object is necessary for well-being

**Psychosis**—psychological state in which the ability to recognize reality, communicate, and relate to others is seriously impaired

**Psychosurgery**—surgical interruption of neural pathways in the brain associated with transmission of emotional impulses

**Psychotic behavior**—severely dysfunctional behavior characterized by panic anxiety, personality disintegration, and regressive behavior

**Rational-emotive therapy**—therapy that focuses on risk taking and on assuming responsibility for one's behavior

**Reaction formation**—use of behaviors that are opposite to what one would like to do

**Reality therapy**—therapy that focuses on recognition and accomplishment of life goals, emphasizing development of capacity to care about self and others

**Relationship therapy** — one-on-one nurse-client relationship in which the nursing process is used to meet the client's needs

**Resistance** — tendency to maintain maladaptive behaviors despite therapeutic intervention

**Role clarification** — gaining of knowledge in order to perform a specific role

**Role modeling** — performing a certain role in a manner that warrants emulation

**Role playing** — acting out a situation in order to deepen one's ability to see from another point of view

**Role reversal** — acting out the role of another person with whom one is in conflict

**Rumination** — persistent thinking about and discussion of a particular idea or subject

**Schizoaffective disorder** — medical diagnosis that denotes symptoms of schizophrenia coupled with an altered mood (usually depression)

**Seclusion** — placement of an agitated client alone in a single room (sometimes locked) to decrease stimuli and to allow the client time to regain control

**Secondary prevention** — actions taken to reduce the prevalence of disease

**Self-actualization** — fulfilling one's potential

**Self-awareness** — recognition of what one experiences and how one reacts to the experiences

**Self-concept** — all knowledge and beliefs held about oneself in relation to one's physical and social environment

**Self-esteem** — feelings held about oneself in relation to personal worth and value

**Semantic fallacies** — misperceptions, distortions, and irrational beliefs that contribute to automatic negative thinking, commonly present in depressed clients

**Somatic therapies** — treatments that affect physiological functioning, such as psychosurgery, electroconvulsive therapy, pharmacotherapy

**Somatoform disorders**—disorders characterized by recurrent and multiple physical symptoms that have no organic or physiologic base

**Stressors**—stimuli that one perceives as challenging, threatening, or demanding; may be pleasant or unpleasant, internal or external, physiologic or psychosocial

**Superego**—mental structure in psychoanalytic theory that evaluates actions of the ego

**Supportive confrontation**—technique used to make a client aware of incongruences in attitudes, feelings, or behaviors by verbalizing observed discrepancies

**Symbolization**—defense mechanism in which an abstract representation is made of an actual object

**Tangentiality**—form of speech, common in schizophrenics, in which the response to a question begins appropriately but then deviates from the topic to related matters

**Tertiary prevention**—actions taken to reduce disability associated with disease

**Therapeutic touch**—Laying a hand on or close to the body of an ill person for the purpose of healing

**Token economy system**—a form of behavior modification in which an object is used as positive reinforcement to promote behavioral change

**Tolerance**—state characterized by the need for increasingly larger doses of a drug to obtain the effects previously obtained at lower doses

**Transference**—projection of feelings about significant others onto the therapist

**Transmethylation**—molecular transformation of one catecholamine to another

**Uncomplicated grief reaction**—healthy, adaptive response to loss; resolved when the lost person or object is internalized, the bonds of attachment are loosened, and new relationships are established

**Undoing**—use of an act or utterance to negate, at least partially, a previous act or utterance

**Violence**—extreme force or destructive action that injures or hurts others

**Visualization** — use of positive mental images to consciously program a desired change

**Withdrawal syndrome** — collection of symptoms that occur after cessation of an abused substance

**Word salad** — communication pattern characterized by a jumble of disconnected words

## B: Answers to Study Questions

### CHAPTER 1

1. The behavioral model is based on the concept that all behavior is learned.

2. In the existential model, the therapist and the client are equals, with the therapist acting as a guide.

3. The six phases of interpersonal development are infancy (ages 1 to 2), childhood (ages 2 to 6), juvenile (ages 6 to 9), preadolescence (ages 9 to 12), early adolescence (ages 12 to 15), and late adolescence (ages 15 to 21).

4. The medical model uses the *Diagnostic and Statistical Manual of Mental Disorders, Third Edition-Revised* (*DSM-III-R*) of the American Psychiatric Association to record and classify diagnoses.

5. Nursing models focus on the client's biological, psychological, and sociocultural needs and on the nurse's caring functions.

6. Sigmund Freud is considered the father of the psychoanalytic model.

7. In the social model, the client initiates therapy and defines the problem. The therapist collaborates with the client to promote change, while advocating freedom of choice and community mental health.

### CHAPTER 2

1. During the late 1800s and early 1900s, nursing care focused on providing custodial care, meeting the client's physical needs, dispensing medications, assisting with hydrotherapy, and encouraging client participation in ward activities.

2. The National Mental Health Act of 1946 created the NIMH.

3. During the 1960s and 1970s, treatment for mentally ill persons moved from institutions to the community.

4. The ANA defines the psychiatric nursing role as a specialized area of nursing practice that employs theories of human behavior as its science and the "powerful use of self" as its art.

5. In primary prevention, psychiatric nursing functions include health education, improvement of socioeconomic conditions, consumer education about normal growth and development, referral before symptoms develop, support of family members, and community and political activity.

6. Psychiatric nurse generalists are baccalaureate prepared. They meet the profession's standards of knowledge, experience, and quality of care. Specialists have graduate education, supervised clinical experience, and a depth of knowledge, competence, and skill in practice.

## CHAPTER 3

1. Stress is a state of imbalance within an organism brought about by an actual or perceived disparity between environmental demands (called stressors) and the organism's capacity to cope with them.

2. The stress response is influenced by the intensity and duration of the stressful stimulus and by the person's perception of control over the stimulus.

3. The three phases of general adaptation syndrome are alarm, resistance, and exhaustion.

4. *DSM-III-R* medical diagnoses and NANDA nursing diagnoses are used to identify stress and psychobiologic disorders.

5. Stress management strategies include progressive relaxation, biofeedback, meditation, hypnosis, guided imagery, behavior modification, yoga, exercise and stretching, attitudinal restructuring, autogenic training, stress desensitization, massage, therapeutic touch, psychotherapy, nutrition, laughter, play, and music.

## CHAPTER 4

1. The five stages of coping with an anticipated death are denial, anger, bargaining, depression, and acceptance.

2. Nursing care goals focus on helping the client to live more fully and comfortably until death, supporting the family, and promoting acceptance of death.

3. The three phases of uncomplicated grief are shock and disbelief; heightened awareness; and reorganization, letting go, and resolution.

4. Symptoms of grief include somatic distress, preoccupation with the deceased, guilt and hostility, and personality disorganization.

5. The nurse sets goals according to the client's needs, then directs interventions toward specific behaviors.

## CHAPTER 5

1. A person's self-concept includes body image, identity, roles, self-esteem, and self-ideals.

2. The three behavioral categories associated with an altered self-concept are low self-esteem, identity confusion, and depersonalization.

3. The primary nursing goals for a client with an altered self-concept are to increase the client's self-realization and self-acceptance while helping the client demonstrate increased confidence and self-worth.

4. When assisting the client with self-evaluation, the nurse should help identify relevant stressors, unrealistic goals, faulty perceptions, strengths, coping

resources, and maladaptive responses. To accomplish this, the nurse can use such techniques as facilitative communication, supportive confrontation, role clarification, and psychodrama.

## CHAPTER 6

1. Freud viewed primary anxiety as a traumatic state that is first produced by external forces during birth. Subsequent anxiety results from the emotional conflict between the primitive impulses of the id and the regulatory function of the superego.

2. A moderate anxiety level focuses one's attention on immediate concerns, narrows the perceptual field, and produces selective inattention.

3. Cardiovascular responses to anxiety include palpitations, tachycardia, changes in blood pressure, and faintness.

4. Affective responses to anxiety include edginess, impatience, uneasiness, tension, fear, and jumpiness.

5. When caring for a client experiencing panic, the nurse must remain calm and try to reduce the client's anxiety.

## CHAPTER 7

1. To be diagnosed with generalized anxiety state, a client must be at least age 18.

2. The key sign of phobia is panic when the client sees the feared object.

3. Key signs and symptoms of a client with an obsessive-compulsive disorder include repetitive thoughts that the person cannot control or exclude from consciousness; recurring, irresistible impulses to perform an action; and defense mechanisms, such as isolation, undoing, reaction formation, and magical thinking.

4. When caring for a client with a post-traumatic stress disorder, the nurse should explore the meaning of the event and assist with problem solving.

5. Nursing interventions for a client with a dissociative disorder should focus on the client and not on the symptoms.

6. Intervention strategies for a client with an anxiety disorder include psychopharmacology, individual psychotherapy, behavior modification, and group therapy.

## CHAPTER 8

1. Biological etiologies for mood disorders include biogenic amine hypothesis, electrolyte metabolism disturbance, neuroendocrine abnormalities, catecholamine imbalance, and a disturbance in biological rhythms.

2. Martin Seligman postulated the learned helplessness concept.

3. Special treatment measures for mood disorders include electroconvulsive therapy, antidepressant medications, lithium therapy, group and individual therapies, phototherapy, and sleep manipulation.

4. Cognitive changes for a client experiencing moderate depression include slow thinking and a narrowing of interests, indecisiveness, self-doubt, rumination, and pessimism.

5. The critical nursing intervention is to assess the depressed client's suicide risk.

6. Nursing care goals for a manic client include preventing the client from self-harm; decreasing disorientation, delusions, bizarre behavior and dress, sexual acting-out, hyperactivity, restlessness and agitation; promoting rest and sleep; providing a nutritious diet; assisting with activities of daily living; providing emotional support; and promoting medication compliance.

## CHAPTER 9

1. High-risk groups include alcoholics; police officers; physicians; those with previous suicide attempts; adolescents; accident repeaters; those who reject treatment; members of minority groups; psychotics; and elderly, terminally ill, or medically ignored persons.

2. Three pharmacologic agents used to treat suicidal clients are antidepressants, antianxiety agents, and antimanic agents.

3. The nurse would determine the appropriate level of suicide precautions and explain them to the client; assess suicide potential daily; re-evaluate the level of precautions daily; obtain assessment data in a matter-of-fact manner; ask the client directly about the suicide plan; remove dangerous objects from the area; place the client in a room near the nurses' station, in view of staff; make sure windows are locked; and stay close to the client when sharp objects must be used.

4. Family nursing care goals and interventions include lessening the long-term effects of grieving and promoting grieving; recognizing that support from friends may be lacking; helping the family explore their guilt; being alert to "anniversary suicide" by relatives; and helping the family deal with hostility and destructiveness.

## CHAPTER 10

1. Psychotic behavior includes various symptoms resulting from disturbed thought process, distorted perceptions, brain damage, or chemical toxicity.

2. The sequential steps of schizophrenia are inability to trust, dissociation, displacement, fantasy, and projection.

3. Primary manifestations of schizophrenia include associative looseness, autistic thinking, ambivalence, and alterations of affect.

4. Hallucinations develop in three phases: the client focuses on comforting thoughts to relieve anxiety and stress; experiences outward projection; and experiences increasing preoccupation and helplessness. The hallucination is controlling but comforting, although content may become menacing.

5. Behavioral manifestations of schizophrenia include withdrawal, regression, overactivity or underactivity, impulsivity, mannerisms, automatism, and stereotypy.

6. The priority problem with a client in an acute psychotic episode relates to basic physical and safety needs.

7. Principles of therapeutic interaction include acceptance of the client, acknowledgment, authenticity, and self-awareness.

8. To help the client establish ego boundaries, the nurse would validate a client's real perceptions and correct misconceptions matter-of-factly; avoid arguing; stay with a frightened client; discuss simple, concrete topics; and provide activities that help the client maintain contact with reality.

## CHAPTER 11

1. Characteristics of healthy interpersonal relationships include intimacy while maintaining separate identities; sensitivity to others' needs; mutual validation of personal worth; open communication of feelings; acceptance of others as valued, separate people; deep, empathic understanding; willingness and ability to subordinate individual needs to the needs of others or to the demands of the relationship; interdependency; and ego-syntony.

2. The young adult forms interdependent relationships, makes independent decisions, implements occupational plans, balances dependent and independent behaviors, and shows increased sensitivity to the feelings and needs of others.

3. Interventions for dependency and helplessness include anticipating the client's needs before they demand attention; setting realistic limits; helping the client manage anxiety; teaching the client to express ideas and feelings assertively; supporting the client in accepting increased decision making; and clarifying roles.

4. The key characteristic of a client experiencing suspiciousness is an inability to trust.

5. An inability to form warm, tender relationships is a hallmark of withdrawal.

6. Treatment modalities for a client with a personality disorder may include, antianxiety medications, behavior modification, and individual psychotherapy.

## CHAPTER 12

1. Behavioral patterns of a substance abuser include dysfunctional anger, manipulation, impulsiveness, avoidance, and grandiosity.

2. Predisposing psychological factors of substance abuse include a dependent personality, low self-esteem, anger and frustration, feelings of omnipotence, depression, and defense mechanisms.

3. In the pre-alcoholic phase, the person uses alcohol to relax and begins to build a tolerance. In the early alcoholic phase, the person sneaks drinks, denies drinking, and blacks out. In the addiction phase, the person loses control over drinking, displays aggressive behavior, blames others for altered relationships, and has withdrawal symptoms. In the chronic phase, the person indulges in unplanned sprees, engages in solitary drinking, and suffers physical complications.

4. During withdrawal, the nurse should monitor vital signs and observe for signs of seizures and impending withdrawal syndrome.

5. Problems during the rehabilitative stage of alcoholism include denial of the illness, failure to understand the disease, low self-esteem, loneliness, low tolerance for frustration, and the possibility of relapse.

6. Behaviors associated with inhalant abuse include euphoria, decreased inhibition, misperceptions or illusions, clouding of thought, drowsiness, and rapidly developed tolerance. No withdrawal symptoms appear.

7. Problems during an acute drug reaction include decreased circulatory and respiratory function, signs of impending withdrawal, potential for self-injury, panic and flashback reactions, and poor nutritional status.

8. The nurse can intervene during denial by focusing on the problem, avoiding the client's attempts to focus on external problems, identifying projection of blame or defensiveness, and avoiding discussion of unanswerable questions.

## CHAPTER 13

1. Functional anger energizes behavior to avoid anxiety, characterizes a healthy relationship, can project a positive self-concept, serves as an ego defense, gives a sense of control, provides immediate relief, and can indicate the need for more effective coping behaviors. Dysfunctional anger arises when early conflicts are reenacted and become a source of tension; it is cyclical and stems from or results in unresolved anger and anxiety, offensive behaviors, powerlessness, and angry responses or rejection by others.

2. Anger can be expressed externally through constructive criticism or aggression.

3. Nursing goals for an angry client include establishing a hierarchy of behaviors while reinforcing mastery and self-control.

4. The nurse would evaluate the client's behavioral changes, subjective responses, appropriateness of expressions of anger, use of assertive behaviors, and problem-solving skills.

## CHAPTER 14

1. Violence carries a physical, emotional, or moral force; arouses fear in others; creates anxiety in victims; and poses a threat to safety. It may be displayed deliberately or may follow a loss of control over aggressive impulses.

2. When intervening with a physically aggressive client, the nurse should take precautions for personal safety and not handle the client alone; approach the client calmly and firmly; use short, concise statements; inform the client what is expected; provide medication; arrange for the seclusion of the client.

3. Motivations for sexual assault include an act of aggression; a means of gaining control; and a desire to humiliate, defile, or dominate the victim.

4. After collecting evidence in a sexual assault case, the nurse should label it carefully in the presence of a witness.

## CHAPTER 15

1. Abuse comprises acts of misuse, exploitation, or deceit intended to injure, damage, maltreat, or corrupt.

2. Family violence comprises physical abuse, neglect, psychological unavailability, verbal hostility, and sexual abuse.

3. Characteristics of a violent family system include closed boundaries; a painful and desperate mood; competition for affection, attention, and nurturance; inability of members to define themselves as individuals apart from the family system; an inability to trust; conflict within the family system; a lack of impulse control and self-discipline; a reduced capacity to delay gratification; inadequate task performance; mixed or double message communication; imbalanced power ratio; and role stereotyping.

4. Behavioral cues for child abuse include wariness of adults, rapid adaptation to the hospital unit, unwillingness to turn to parents for support, abnormal eating or drinking habits, excessive crying or none at all, and extreme fear of or total lack of respect for authority figures.

5. The nurse's self-awareness is essential for intervention.

## CHAPTER 16

1. Crisis occurs when stress overwhelms the individual's usual coping mechanisms. It is self-limiting, typically resolving within 6 weeks.

2. Crisis intervention increases the likelihood that a crisis will be positively resolved, offers immediate help and reestablishes equilibrium, can restore the client's precrisis level of functioning, and teaches the client effective problem-solving skills.

3. In the therapeutic environment, the nurse acts primarily in inpatient settings to facilitate and oversee implementation of interventions, to act as a role model, and to structure the client's environment.

4. Membership roles in groups include task roles, maintenance roles, and egocentric roles.

5. The focus of family therapy is on family interaction.

6. The clinical nurse specialist acts as a psychotherapist in uncovering therapy; the nurse generalist acts as a supportive therapist, counseling the client and maintaining the nurse-client relationship.

7. Biological therapies focus on symptoms, diagnoses, and prognoses.

## C: ANA Classification of Human Responses of Concern for Psychiatric Mental Health Nursing Practice

The following classification is based on previous work of the Phenomenon Task Force and the Advisory Panel on Classifications for Nursing Practice of the American Nurses' Association. Asterisks indicate a NANDA diagnosis.

01. Human response patterns in activity processes
  01.01 Altered motor behavior
    01.01.01 Bizarre motor behavior
    01.01.02 Catatonia
    01.01.03 Impaired coordination
    01.01.04 Hyperactivity
    01.01.05 Hypoactivity
    01.01.06 Muscular rigidity
    01.01.07 Psychomotor retardation
  01.02 Altered recreation patterns
    01.02.01 Inadequate diversional activity
  01.03 Altered self-care
    01.03.01 Altered eating
    *01.03.02 Altered grooming
    01.03.03 Altered health maintenance
    *01.03.04 Altered hygiene
    01.03.05 Altered participation in health care
    *01.03.06 Altered toileting
  01.04 Altered sleep/arousal patterns
    01.04.01 Difficult transition to and from sleep
    01.04.02 Hypersomnia
    01.04.03 Insomnia
    01.04.04 Nightmares
    01.04.05 Somnolence
  01.97 Undeveloped activity processes
  01.98 Altered activity processes not otherwise specified
  01.99 Potential for altered activity/processes

02. Human response patterns in cognition processes
  02.01 Altered decision making
  02.02 Altered judgment
  *02.03 Altered knowledge processes
    02.03.01 Agnosia
    02.03.02 Altered intellectual functioning
    *02.03.03 Knowledge deficit
  02.04 Altered learning processes
  02.05 Altered memory
    02.05.01 Amnesia
    02.05.02 Distorted memory
    02.05.03 Long-term memory loss
    02.05.04 Short-term memory loss
  02.06 Altered orientation
    02.06.01 Confusion
    02.06.02 Delirium
    02.06.03 Disorientation
  02.07 Altered thought content
    02.07.01 Delusions
    02.07.02 Ideas of reference
    02.07.03 Magical thinking
    02.07.04 Obsessions

(continued)

## A.N.A. CLASSIFICATION OF HUMAN RESPONSES OF CONCERN FOR PSYCHIATRIC MENTAL HEALTH NURSING PRACTICE (continued)

*02.08 Altered thought processes
02.08.01 Altered abstract
thinking
02.08.02 Altered concentration
02.08.03 Altered problem
solving
02.08.04 Thought insertion
02.97 Undeveloped cognition
processes
02.98 Altered cognition processes
not otherwise specified
02.99 Potential for altered
cognition processes

---

03. Human response patterns in
ecological processes
03.01 Altered community
maintenance
03.01.01 Community safety
hazards
03.01.02 Community sanitation
hazards
03.02 Altered environmental
integrity
*03.03 Altered home maintenance
03.03.01 Home safety hazards
03.03.02 Home sanitation
hazards

---

04. Human response patterns in
emotional processes
04.01 Abuse response patterns
*04.01.01 Rape-trauma
syndrome
04.02 Altered feeling patterns
04.02.01 Anger
*04.02.02 Anxiety
04.02.03 Elation
04.02.04 Envy

*04.02.05 Fear
*04.02.06 Grief
04.02.07 Guilt
04.02.08 Sadness
04.02.09 Shame
04.03 Undifferentiated feeling
pattern
04.97 Undeveloped emotional
responses
04.98 Altered emotional processes
not otherwise specified
04.99 Potential for altered
emotional processes

---

05. Human response patterns in
interpersonal processes
*05.01 Altered communication
processes
05.01.01 Altered nonverbal
communication
*05.01.02 Altered verbal
communication
05.02 Altered conduct/impulse
processes
05.02.01 Aggressive/violent
behaviors
05.02.01.01 Aggressive/vio-
lent behaviors
toward environ-
ment
05.02.01.02 Aggressive/vio-
lent behaviors
toward others
05.02.01.03 Aggressive/vio-
lent behaviors
toward self

## A.N.A. CLASSIFICATION OF HUMAN RESPONSES OF CONCERN FOR PSYCHIATRIC MENTAL HEALTH NURSING PRACTICE (continued)

05.02.02 Dysfunctional behaviors
05.02.02.01 Age-inappropriate behaviors
05.02.02.02 Bizarre behaviors
05.02.02.03 Compulsive behaviors
05.02.02.04 Disorganized behaviors
05.02.02.05 Unpredictable behaviors
05.03 Altered role performance
05.03.01 Altered family role
05.03.02 Altered leisure role
*05.03.03 Altered parenting role
05.03.04 Altered play role
05.03.05 Altered student role
05.03.06 Altered work role
05.04 Altered sexuality processes
05.05 Altered social interaction
05.05.01 Social intrusiveness
*05.05.02 Social isolation/withdrawal
05.97 Undeveloped interpersonal processes
05.98 Altered interpersonal processes not otherwise specified
05.99 Potential for altered interpersonal processes
*05.99.01 Potential for violence

06. Human response patterns in perception processes
06.01 Altered attention
06.01.01 Distractibility
06.01.02 Hyperalertness
06.01.03 Inattention
06.01.04 Selective attention

*06.02 Altered comfort patterns
06.02.01 Discomfort
06.02.02 Distress
06.02.03 Pain
06.03 Altered self-concept
*06.03.01 Altered body image
06.03.02 Altered gender identity
*06.03.03 Altered personal identity
*06.03.04 Altered self-esteem
06.03.05 Altered social identity
06.03.06 Undeveloped self-concept
06.04 Altered sensory perception
*06.04.01 Auditory
*06.04.02 Gustatory
06.04.03 Hallucinations
06.04.04 Illusions
*06.04.05 Kinesthetic
*06.04.06 Olfactory
*06.04.07 Tactile
*06.04.08 Visual
06.97 Undeveloped perception processes
06.98 Altered perception processes not otherwise specified
06.99 Potential for altered perception processes

07. Human response patterns in physiological processes
07.01 Altered circulation processes
07.01.01 Altered vascular circulation
*07.01.01.01 Tissue perfusion
*07.01.01.02 Altered fluid volume
07.01.02 Altered cardiac circulation

(continued)

**A.N.A. CLASSIFICATION OF HUMAN RESPONSES OF CONCERN FOR PSYCHIATRIC MENTAL HEALTH NURSING PRACTICE** (continued)

07.02 Altered elimination
    processes
  *07.02.01 Altered bowel
    elimination
    *07.02.01.01 Constipation
    *07.02.01.02 Diarrhea
    *07.02.01.03 Incontinence
    07.02.01.04 Encopresis
  *07.02.02 Altered urinary
    elimination
    *07.02.02.01 Incontinence
    *07.02.02.02 Retention
    07.02.02.03 Enuresis
  07.02.03 Altered skin
    elimination
07.03 Altered endocrine/metabolic
    processes
  07.03.01 Altered growth
  07.03.02 Altered hormone
    regulation
    07.03.02.01 Premenstrual
      stress syndrome
07.04 Altered gastrointestinal
    processes
  07.04.01 Altered absorption
  07.04.02 Altered digestion
07.05 Altered neurosensory
    processes
  07.05.01 Altered levels of
    consciousness
  07.05.02 Altered sensory acuity
  07.05.03 Altered sensory
    processing
  07.05.04 Altered sensory
    integration
    07.05.04.01 Learning
      disabilities

07.06 Altered nutrition processes
  07.06.01 Altered cellular
    processes
  07.06.02 Altered systemic
    processes
    *07.06.02.01 More than body
      requirements
    *07.06.02.02 Less than body
      requirements
  07.06.03 Altered eating
    processes
    07.06.03.01 Anorexia
    07.06.03.02 Pica
07.07 Altered oxygenation
    processes
  07.07.01 Altered respiration
    07.07.01.01 Altered gas
      exchange
    *07.07.01.02 Ineffective air-
      way clearance
    *07.07.01.03 Ineffective
      breathing
      pattern
07.08 Altered physical integrity
    processes
  *07.08.01 Altered skin integrity
  *07.08.02 Altered tissue
    integrity
07.09 Altered physical regulation
    processes
  07.09.01 Altered immune
    responses
    07.09.01.01 Infection
07.10 Altered body temperature
  *07.10.01 Hypothermia
  *07.10.02 Hyperthermia
  *07.10.03 Ineffective
    thermoregulation

## A.N.A. CLASSIFICATION OF HUMAN RESPONSES OF CONCERN FOR PSYCHIATRIC MENTAL HEALTH NURSING PRACTICE *(continued)*

07.97 Undeveloped physiological
      processes
07.98 Altered physiological
      processes not otherwise
      specified
07.99 Potential for altered
      physiological processes

08. Human response patterns in
    valuation processes
*08.01 Altered meaningfulness
  *08.01.01 Hopelessness
  08.01.02 Helplessness
  08.01.03 Loneliness
  *08.01.04 Powerlessness
08.02 Altered Spirituality
  *08.02.01 Spiritual distress
  08.02.02 Spiritual despair
08.03 Altered values
  08.03.01 Conflict with social
         order
  08.03.02 Inability to
         internalize values
  08.03.03 Unclarified values
08.97 Undeveloped valuation
      processes
08.98 Altered valuation processes
      not otherwise specified
08.99 Potential for altered
      valuation processes

From M. Loomis, et al. *ANA Classification of Individual Human Responses.* American Nurses' Association, 1986. Used with permission.

# Selected References

Beck, C.M., et al. *Mental Health–Psychiatric Nursing: A Holistic Life-Cycle Approach*, 2nd ed. St. Louis: C.V. Mosby Co., 1988.

Burgess, A.W. *Psychiatric Nursing in the Hospital and Community*, 5th ed. Norwalk, Conn.: Appleton & Lange, 1990.

Gary, F., and Kavanagh, C.K. *Psychiatric Mental Health Nursing*. Philadelphia: J.B. Lippincott Co., 1991.

Haber, J., et al. *Comprehensive Psychiatric Nursing*, 4th ed. St. Louis: C.V. Mosby Co., 1987.

Janosik, E.H., and Davies, J.L. *Psychiatric Mental Health Nursing*, 2nd ed. Boston: Jones & Bartlett Pubs., 1989.

Johnson, B.S. *Psychiatric–Mental Health Nursing*, 2nd ed. Philadelphia: J.B. Lippincott Co., 1989.

McFarland, G.K., and Thomas, M.D. *Psychiatric Mental Health Nursing: Application of the Nursing Process*. Philadelphia: J.B. Lippincott Co., 1991.

Norris, J., et al. *Mental Health–Psychiatric Nursing: A Continuum of Care*. New York: John Wiley & Sons, 1987.

Schultz, J.M., and Dark, S.L. *Manual of Psychiatric Care Plans*, 3rd ed. Philadelphia: J.B. Lippincott Co., 1990.

Stuart, G.W., and Sundeen, S.J. *Principles and Practice of Psychiatric Nursing*, 4th ed. St. Louis: Mosby-Year Book, Inc., 1991.

Wilson, H.S., and Kneisl, C.R. *Psychiatric Nursing*, 3rd ed. Menlo Park, Calif: Addison-Wesley Publishing Co., 1988.

# Index

**A**

Abuse
domestic
behavioral cues to, 128, 155
categories of, 125, 132
characteristics of, 126-128, 132, 155
definitions of, 125, 132
diagnoses for (medical and nursing), 128-129
epidemiology of, 126
etiology of, 126
nursing interventions for, 129, 132, 155
physical symptoms of, 128
treatments for, 129-130
substance. See Alcoholism; Drug abuse.
Adaptation, 4, 142
Addiction, 142. See also Alcoholism; Drug abuse.
Affect, 56, 79, 142
Aggression, 109, 123, 142, 154, 155
characteristics of, 116
theories of, 57, 116
Alcoholism
behaviors associated with, 96, 99-100, 107
diagnoses for (medical and nursing), 98-99
hallucinosis and, 100
nursing interventions for
acute stage, 100-101
rehabilitative stage, 101, 107, 154
predisposing factors in, 96-97
Alienation, 48, 142
American Nurses' Association (ANA), 11, 17, 149
Standards of Psychiatric and Mental Health Nursing Practice, 13t-14t, 15
American Psychiatric Association, 4

Anger
assessment of, 110-111
characteristics of, 109
diagnoses for (medical and nursing), 111-112
dysfunctional, 109, 114, 154
expressions of, 109-110
functional, 109, 114, 154
nursing interventions for, 112, 114, 154
precipitating stressors in, 110
Anticipatory guidance, 29, 142
Antidepressants, 58, 152
Antisocial personality disorder, 91
Anxiety, 3
affective responses to, 43, 151
behavioral responses to, 42
characteristics of, 40
cognitive responses to, 42-43
coping strategies for, 43
levels of, 41
nursing interventions for, 43-44, 46, 151
physiologic responses to, 41-42, 46, 151
precipitating stressors in, 40-41
theories on, 40, 151
Anxiety-related disorders
characteristics of, 48
dissociative disorders, 51, 54, 151
generalized anxiety state, 48-49, 54, 151
nursing interventions for, 51-52, 151
obsessive-compulsive disorder, 49-50, 54, 151
phobias, 49, 54, 151
post-traumatic stress disorder, 50, 54, 120, 151
somatoform disorders, 50-51, 147
Assaultive behavior. See Abuse, domestic; Aggression; Sexual assault; Violence.
Attitudinal restructuring, 21, 142
Autistic thinking, 77-78, 142
Autogenic training, 21, 142
Aversion therapy, 2, 142

**B**
Beck, Aaron, 57
Behavioral model, 2, 8, 57, 149
Behavior modification, 52, 105, 142, 151
Biofeedback, 21, 142
Biogenic model, 4
Biological therapies, 139, 141, 156
Bipolar affective disorder, 56, 58
Body image, 33, 142
    alterations in, 79
Borderline personality disorder, 91
Bowlby, J., 57

**C**
Caplan, Gerald, 6
Carbamazepine, 58
Child abuse, 126, 132, 155
Clang association, 78, 142
Clinical nurse specialist, 139, 141, 156
Cognitive model, 57
Community mental health, 6, 142, 149
Community Mental Health Act (1963),
    10
Consensual validation, 90, 142
Conversion disorder, 50-51, 143
Coping mechanisms, 27, 143, 150
Counter-conditioning, 2, 143
Crisis intervention, 12, 120, 129, 134-
    135, 141, 143

**D**
Death
    coping stages of, 26, 31, 150
    emotional responses to, 26
    nursing interventions for, 26-27, 31,
        150
Defense mechanisms, 43, 143, 151
Degenerative dementia, 69, 143
Delayed grief reactions, 28
Delusions, 78, 83, 143
Dependency, 89-90, 93, 153
Depersonalization, 51, 143
Depressant abuse, 102
Depression, 56, 59-61, 64, 143
Desensitization, 2, 21, 143
*Diagnostic and Statistical Manual of
    Mental Disorders (DSM-III-R)*, 4,
    149
Dichotomous thinking, 68, 143

Disorders, kinds of
    antisocial personality, 91
    anxiety-related, 48-54, 151
    bipolar affective, 56, 58
    borderline personality, 91
    conversion, 50-51, 143
    dissociative, 51, 54, 151
    mood, 56-64, 152
    obsessive-compulsive, 49-50, 54, 151
    paranoid personality, 89, 90
    personality, 89-93, 153
    post-traumatic stress, 50, 54, 120, 151
    schizoaffective, 69, 146
    schizoid personality, 90
    schizotypal personality, 90
    somatoform, 50-51, 147
    unipolar affective, 56, 58
Dissociative disorders, 51, 54, 151
Distorted grief reactions, 28, 31
Dopamine hypothesis, 77
Drug abuse
    behaviors associated with, 101-103
    common drugs in, 97-98
    consequences of, 103-104
    diagnoses for (medical and nursing),
        98-99
    nursing interventions for
        acute stage, 104, 107, 154
        rehabilitative stage, 104-105, 107
    predisposing factors in, 97-98

**E**
Echolalia, 78, 143
Ectomorph, 4
Ego boundaries, 79, 82, 86, 153
Ego-dystonic behavior, 48, 143
Ego-syntonic behavior, 88, 143
Elder abuse, 126
Electroconvulsive therapy, 58, 139, 152
Ellis, Albert, 2
Empathy, 88, 143
Encounter group therapy, 2, 143
Endomorph, 4
Erikson, Eric, 6
Exhibitionism, 125, 144
Existentialism, 2, 137, 144
Existential model, 2-3, 8, 149

**F**
Family therapy, 81, 137-138, 141, 156
Feedback, 90, 144
Fight-or-flight response, 19, 144
Free association, 6, 144
Freud, Anna, 6
Freud, Sigmund, 5, 40, 46, 57, 149, 151
Fromm-Reichman, Freida, 6

**G**
General adaptation syndrome, 19, 20, 24, 150
Generalized anxiety state, 48-49, 54, 151
Gestalt therapy, 2, 144
Glasser, William, 2
Grieving, 144
  nursing interventions for, 28-29, 150
  symptoms of, 27-28, 31, 150
  types of, 28, 150
Group therapy, 52, 58, 81, 105, 136-137, 141, 151, 152, 156
Guidance, anticipatory, 29, 142
Guided imagery, 21, 144

**H**
Hallucinations, 79, 83, 86, 153
Hallucinogen abuse, 102-103
Heidegger, Martin, 2
Helplessness, 89-90, 93, 153
  learned, 57, 64, 151
Holism, 4, 144
Horney, Karen, 6
Hostility, 110, 144
Hypochondriasis, 50-51, 144

**I-J**
Id, 40, 144, 151
Identity, 33, 144
Illness, prevention of
  primary, 12, 145, 149
  secondary, 12, 146
  tertiary, 14, 147
Imagery, guided, 21, 144
Impulsivity, 91, 93
Incest, 125, 144
Inhalant abuse, 103, 107, 154
Interpersonal model, 3, 4, 8, 149

**K**
Kierkegaard, Soren, 2
King, Imogene, 4
Klein, Melanie, 6

**L**
Laing, R.D., 2
Learned helplessness, 57, 64, 151
Lewinsohn, P., 57
Lithium, 58, 152

**M**
Magical thinking, 49, 144, 151
Mania, 56, 61-62, 64, 144, 152
Manipulation, 91, 93
Marijuana abuse, 103
Medical model, 3-4, 8, 149
Menninger, Karl, 6
Mental Health Survey Act (1955), 10
Mental Health Systems Act (1980), 10, 11
Milieu, 12, 144
  therapy, 10, 81, 136, 144
Models, conceptual
  behavioral, 2, 8, 57, 149
  biogenic, 4
  existential, 2-3, 8, 149
  interpersonal, 3, 4, 8, 149
  medical, 3-4, 8, 149
  nursing, 4-5, 8, 149
  psychoanalytic, 5-6, 8, 149
  self-care, 4
  social, 6, 8, 149
  systems, 4
Mood disorders
  classification of, 56
  depressive reactions in, 59-61, 152
  diagnoses for (medical and nursing), 58-59
  epidemiology of, 57-58
  etiology of, 56-57, 64, 151
  manic reactions in, 61-62, 152
  treatments for, 58, 64, 152
Multiple personality, 51
Mutism, 78, 145

**N**
National Institute of Mental Health (NIMH), 10, 11, 17, 149
National Mental Health Act (1946), 10, 149
National Mental Health Leadership Forum, 11
Neglect, 125
Neologism, 78, 145
Neurotic behavior, 5, 145

North American Nursing Diagnosis Association (NANDA), 5
Nurse generalist, 139, 141, 149, 156
Nursing models, 4-5, 8, 149

**O**
Object-loss theory, 57
Obsessive-compulsive disorder, 49-50, 54, 151
Operant conditioning, 2, 145
Opiate abuse, 101-102
Orem, Dorothea, 4

**P-Q**
Panic, 41, 46, 151
Paranoid personality disorder, 89, 90
Pavlov, Ivan, 2
Peplau, Hildegarde, 4
Perception, schizophrenia and, 76, 145
Perls, Frederick, 2
Personality disorders
  dependency and helplessness in, 89-90, 93, 153
  impulsivity and manipulation in, 91, 93
  predisposing factors in, 89
  suspiciousness in, 90, 93, 153
  treatments for, 91, 93, 153
  withdrawal in, 90-91, 153
Phobias, 49, 54, 151
Phototherapy, 58, 152
Post-traumatic stress disorder, 50, 54, 120, 151
President's Commission on Mental Health, 10
Projection, 90, 145
Psychiatric nursing
  ANA practice standards for, 13t-14t
  history of, 10-11
  roles and functions of, 11-12, 14t, 17
  treatments used in, 134-139
Psychoanalytic model, 5-6, 8, 149
Psychodrama, 36, 137, 145, 151
Psychogenic amnesia, 51
Psychogenic fugue, 51, 145
Psychogenic pain, 50, 145
Psychopharmacology, 51, 81, 151
Psychosexual development, 5-6
Psychosis, 67, 145
Psychosurgery, 4, 139, 145

Psychotherapy, 58, 81, 105, 138-139, 141, 151, 152
Psychotic behavior, 6, 76, 80, 86, 145, 152, 153

**R**
Rape. *See* Sexual assault.
Rational-emotive therapy, 2, 145
Reaction formation, 49, 145, 151
Reality therapy, 2, 145
Relatedness, 88-89, 93
Relationships, interpersonal, 88, 93, 153
Relationship therapy, 81, 146
Resistance, 89, 146
Restructuring, attitudinal, 21, 142
Robertson, J., 57
Rogers, Carl, 2
Rogers, Martha, 4
Role
  clarification, 36, 146, 151
  modeling, 36, 146
  playing, 36, 146
  reversal, 36, 146
Roy, Sister Callista, 4
Rumination, 71, 111, 146

**S**
Sartre, Jean Paul, 2
Schizoaffective disorder, 69, 146
Schizoid personality disorder, 90
Schizophrenia, 77, 86, 152
  affect and, 79
  body image alterations and, 79
  diagnoses for (medical and nursing), 80-81
  etiology of, 76-77
  hallucinations and, 79, 83, 86, 153
  manifestations of
    behavioral, 79-80, 86, 153
    cognitive, 78
    linguistic, 78
    primary, 77-78, 86, 152
    social, 80
  nursing interventions for, 81-83
  treatments for, 81, 153
Schizotypal personality disorder, 90
Seclusion, 118, 146
Self-actualization, 34, 146
Self-awareness, 36, 146
Self-care model, 4

Self-concept, 40, 146, 150
  alterations in
    behaviors associated with, 34-35, 38,
      150
    diagnoses for (medical and nursing),
      35
    nursing interventions for, 35-36, 38,
      150
  components of, 33-34, 38
  healthy personality and, 34
Self-esteem, 33-34, 146
Seligman, Martin, 57, 64, 151
Semantic fallacies, 68, 146
Sexual assault
  assessment of, 119-120
  characteristics of, 119
  diagnoses for (medical and nursing),
    120
  incidence of, 119
  motivations for, 119, 123, 155
  nursing interventions for, 120, 123
  treatments for, 120-121, 155
  victim reactions to, 119
Skinner, B.F., 2
Sleep manipulation, 58, 152
Social model, 6, 8, 149
Social support systems, 105
Somatic therapies, 10, 146
Somatoform disorders, 50-51, 147
Spitz, R., 57
Spouse abuse, 126
Stimulant abuse, 102
Stress, 150
  assessment of, 20
  characteristics of, 19
  diagnoses for (medical and nursing),
    20-21, 24, 150
  illness related to, 19-20
  management strategies for, 21-22, 24,
    150
  nursing interventions for, 21
  physiologic responses to, 19
Stressors, 5, 19, 36, 40-41, 68-69, 110,
    147, 150
Substance abuse. *See* Alcoholism; Drug
    abuse.

Suicidal behavior
  diagnoses for (medical and nursing),
    69-70
  epidemiology of, 66
  high-risk groups for, 67, 74, 152
  myths about, 66
  nursing interventions for, 70-72, 74,
    152
  stressors and risk factors in, 68-69
  theories on, 67
Sullivan, Harry Stack, 3, 10, 40
Superego, 40, 147, 151
Supportive confrontation, 36, 147
Suspiciousness, 90, 93, 153
Symbolization, 49, 147
Systems model, 4
Szasz, Thomas, 6

**T**
Tangentiality, 78, 147
Therapeutic environment, 135-136, 141,
    155
Therapeutic interaction, 81, 86, 153
Therapeutic touch, 22, 147
Therapy, types of
  aversion, 2, 142
  biological, 139, 141, 156
  electroconvulsive, 58, 139, 152
  encounter group, 2, 143
  family, 81, 137-138, 141, 156
  gestalt, 2, 144
  group, 52, 58, 81, 105, 136-137, 141,
    151, 152, 156
  milieu, 10, 81, 136, 144
  phototherapy, 58, 152
  psychotherapy, 58, 81, 105, 138-139,
    141, 151, 152
  rational-emotive, 2, 145
  relationship, 81, 146
  somatic, 10, 146
  *See also* Treatment modalities.
Token economy system, 2, 147
Tolerance, addiction and, 95, 147
Transference, 6, 147
Transmethylation, 4, 76, 147

Treatment modalities
   biological therapies, 139, 141, 156
   crisis intervention, 134-135, 155
   family therapy, 81, 137-138, 141, 156
   group therapy, 52, 58, 81, 105, 136-
      137, 141, 151, 152, 156
   individual psychotherapy, 138-139
   therapeutic environment, 135-136,
      141, 155

**U**
Uncomplicated grief reaction, 26, 31,
   147, 150
Undoing, obsessive-compulsive disorder
   and, 49, 147, 151
Unipolar affective disorder, 56, 58
Unitary Man, 4

**V**
Verbal hostility, 125
Victims, characteristics of, 127-128
Violence, 125, 147
   behavioral cues for, 117
   characteristics of, 116-117, 123, 155
   diagnoses for (medical and nursing),
      117-118
   nursing interventions for, 118
   precipitating factors in, 117
Visualization, 36, 148

**W-X-Y-Z**
Withdrawal
   personality disorders and, 90-91, 153
   substance abuse and, 95, 100, 107,
      148, 154
Wolpe, J., 2
Word salad, 78, 148

t refers to a table.

# Notes

# Notes